Stephen L. Isaacs and
David C. Colby, Editors

Foreword by Risa Lavizzo-Mourey

To Improve Health and Health Care

Volume XV

The Robert Wood Johnson Foundation Anthology

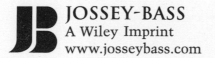

JOSSEY-BASS
A Wiley Imprint
www.josseybass.com

Published by Jossey-Bass
A Wiley Imprint
One Montgomery Street, Suite 1200, San Francisco, CA 94104-4594—-www.josseybass.com

Jossey-Bass books and products are available through most bookstores. To contact Jossey-Bass directly call our Customer Care Department within the U.S. at 800-956-7739, outside the U.S. at 317-572-3986, or fax 317-572-4002.

Wiley also publishes its books in a variety of electronic formats and by print-on-demand. Some material included with standard print versions of this book may not be included in e-books or in print-on-demand. If the version of this book that you purchased references media such as CD or DVD that was not included in your purchase, you may download this material at http://booksupport.wiley.com. For more information about Wiley products, visit www.wiley.com.

ISSN: 1547-3570
ISBN: 978-11184-8814-0

Printed in the United States of America
FIRST EDITION

PB Printing 10 9 8 7 6 5 4 3 2 1

⎯m⎯ Contents

—ᴡ—Foreword

Risa Lavizzo-Mourey

This volume of the *Anthology* marks the fortieth anniversary of the Robert Wood Johnson Foundation as a national philanthropy. In preparing for the commemoration, I reread the oral histories given by the Foundation's original Board and staff members. What struck me about the interviews was the recurrence of two common themes: first, the founders' optimism—their sense that this foundation could make a measurable difference in people's lives; and second, their commitment to upholding the values of Robert Wood Johnson—in particular, his passion to serve the most needy and the most vulnerable individuals.

As I look back over forty years, I think it is fair to say that we have remained faithful to the vision of our original Board and staff. Even though these are difficult times for those of us committed to improving health and health care throughout the United States, I am proud of our legacy and all that we have accomplished. Over the years, as Stephen Isaacs and David Colby point out in their editors' introduction, the Foundation *has* had an impact: occasionally at the policy level, sometimes at the program level, and often at the individual level.

Because this is an anniversary issue, we thought it would be appropriate to offer a comprehensive view of the Foundation and its work over the past four decades. Thus, this volume begins with a brief history of the Foundation—what it has done and how it has evolved—by David Colby, Stephen Isaacs, and Sarah Pickell, followed by some reflections of my own as I complete ten years as the Foundation's fourth president and CEO. The review of the Foundation's first forty years is completed by reprinting six chapters from previous volumes of the *Anthology* that shed light on the way the Foundation works. These include an appreciation of the legendary grantmaker Terry Keenan and chapters on evaluation, communications, national programs, and our New Jersey programs, plus my own "five Cs," where I discuss the various tools beyond making grants that foundations can use to help bring about social change.

The final section of this *Anthology* looks at six current or recently completed programs that have considerable potential significance. Project ECHO is providing access to faraway specialists for primary care physicians dealing with their patients' serious illnesses; The Food Trust is bringing supermarkets to inner cities that lack healthy and nutritious foods; the Health & Society Scholars and the Young Epidemiology Scholars programs have attempted to attract new, younger people to the field of public health; through home- and community-based services, the Connecticut-based Child FIRST program is demonstrating how to decrease developmental and emotional problems in young children; and County Health Rankings & Roadmaps are providing tools on which localities can base efforts to improve the health of their residents.

An anniversary is a time to look forward as well as backward. Despite the many challenges we face and the often discouraging times we live in, I feel quite confident that the work we and our grantees have done since 1972 gives us a solid base on which to move forward. Martin Luther King, Jr. once said, "Change does not roll in on the wheels of inevitability, but comes through continuous struggle." I believe this is true, and that the work of all of us dedicated to making Americans healthier and the health care system fairer will help bring about the change we seek.

—ᴍ—Significant and Long-Lasting Change
Editors' Introduction

Stephen L. Isaacs and David C. Colby

The publication of this *Anthology* volume marking the fortieth anniversary of the Robert Wood Johnson Foundation seemed like a good time to look back and consider where the Foundation has had its greatest impact in improving health and health care—that is, where it has helped bring about significant and long-lasting change—and what elements led to the Foundation's having had that impact. In other words, what are the approaches that characterize the Foundation's work over four decades and have led to the Foundation's effectiveness in areas ranging from tobacco control to emergency medical services and from palliative care to nursing?

The first eight chapters of this *Anthology*—two original contributions and six reprints from past volumes—explore these questions. Taken together, they explore the essence of the Robert Wood Johnson Foundation. The final five chapters present a sampling of current programs and their approaches to addressing specific important problems—such as lack of specialty care in rural areas, unhealthy food choices in inner cities, and building the field of population health research.

Although we are exploring the Foundation's role in bringing about significant and long-lasting change, we should recognize up front that foundations do not generally have the financial firepower to transform any given area by themselves. But by working in concert with others and by using the many tools at their disposal, foundations can play an important and, in some cases, a key role.

Nor do we want to leave the overly rosy impression that the Foundation's first forty years have been characterized by a string of transformational successes. In many areas the Foundation barely made a dent in reaching its priorities—advancing primary care and containing costs are two prime examples. In Volume XIII of the *Anthology*, we wrote about some failures that led to learning opportunities and others that just wasted the Foundation's resources.

No single element explains why some Foundation efforts have a positive impact or even change a field. Sometimes success comes through an influential person taking an interest, circumstances coming together, or simply dumb luck. Successful change is not always—nor even usually—a rational, linear process. But there do seem to be some common elements at play. Among them:

- *Catching the wave*. Before the Foundation became involved in end-of-life care, smoking, and AIDS, there was already interest in improving the care of dying people, smoking was on the decline, and AIDS had become an important health and social concern. Recognizing the trends, the Foundation seized the opportunities, entered the areas, and was able to shape the way they developed.

- *Sticking with important priorities for a long time*. The Robert Wood Johnson Foundation maintained its priority of expanding access to health care for nearly forty years before seeing a major breakthrough in 2010 with the passage of the Affordable Care Act. The Foundation has been dogged in advancing school-based health services for almost as long a period, and improving quality of care has been on its agenda since 1972. Its commitment to nurse-family partnerships has endured for nearly three decades. The Foundation's anti-smoking efforts started in 1991 and continue today. Also dating from the 1980s is its ongoing funding of supportive housing for vulnerable people.

- *Finding, nurturing, and working with outstanding people*. In all, or nearly all, of the successful programs, a handful of individuals who are passionate about the importance of the topic have moved it along. Five obvious examples: Diane Meier in the case of palliative care; Matt Myers in the case of tobacco; John Wennberg in the case of quality; David Olds in the case of nurse-family partnerships; and Edward Wagner in the case of chronic care. It is easy to think in terms of strategies and plans, but individuals make things happen. By supporting those individuals, the Foundation increases the chance of good things happening.

  The Foundation has not merely worked with strong leaders; it has also invested in developing them. Since 1972 the Clinical Scholars and Health Policy Fellows programs have supported researchers and leaders, mainly physicians; since 1992, Scholars in Health Policy Research has developed social science researchers interested in health; and since 2001, Health & Society Scholars, which is discussed in Chapter 11, has invested in researchers interested in the field of population health. These investments have paid off handsomely: foundation presidents, federal agency heads, and academic medical center leaders are products of the Foundation's investments.

- *Taking a wide-ranging approach to a problem and adapting it when appropriate*. In areas as varied as palliative care, tobacco control, access to care, quality, and nursing, the Foundation took a comprehensive approach, using all the tools available to philanthropy: research, advocacy, communications, evaluation, training and fellowships, demonstration programs, and organizational development. And, taking to heart the former

Foundation president and CEO Steven Schroeder's dictum that "execution trumps strategy," the Foundation has not hesitated to adjust its tactics when necessary to achieve its strategic goals.

- *Researching the problem.* Many foundations conduct literature reviews and environmental scans as part of their work. The Robert Wood Johnson Foundation does these as well, but equally significant, it has supported original, sometimes path-breaking research to understand the extent and causes of problems it wants to address, and often to find solutions to them. For example, the Foundation has funded research on access to care, end-of-life care, drug and alcohol use, tobacco taxes, and clean indoor-air laws—to name just a few.

  Moreover, the Foundation has committed long-term funding to organizations that conduct high-quality research on issues of importance to the Foundation—organizations such as Dartmouth University, which produces *The Dartmouth Atlas of Health Care*, and the Center for Studying Health System Change, which monitors changes in health care markets.

- *Evaluating rigorously and communicating strategically.* The Foundation has used two of the tools available to foundations with particular effectiveness: evaluation and communications. Both have been core elements of the Foundation since the beginning. Rigorously evaluating and then sharing results of programs such as nurse-family partnerships, hospice care, and long-term care insurance partnerships, for example, led to their expansion. Active communications programs played an important part in advancing the Foundation's priorities in health insurance expansion, nursing, tobacco, and substance abuse.

- *Remembering and doggedly pursuing the values that the Robert Wood Johnson Foundation stands for.* Its mission—to improve the health and health care of all Americans—not only sets an overall direction for the Foundation; it also provides a moral compass. By keeping the mission in the forefront and developing clear and thoughtful strategies to reach it, the Foundation has been able to maintain its focus on what is really important.

—ᨆ—Acknowledgments

We are immensely grateful to all those who contributed to this volume of the *Anthology*. It was truly a team effort. Carolyn Shea did her usual standout job as fact checker. Jim Morgan, in his first year as copy editor, improved the quality of every chapter. Jim Knickman and Jon Showstack made invaluable suggestions as our outside reviewers. Jamie Bussel, Calvin Bland, Abbey Cofsky, Dee Colello, Rona Henry, Maryjoan Ladden, Jane Lowe, Robin Mockenhaupt, Floyd Morris, Marco Navarro, Steven Schroeder, Polly Seitz, and Beth Toner read and commented on individual chapters or chapter introductions. Ilan Isaacs proofread the entire manuscript before its submission to Jossey-Bass.

At the Robert Wood Johnson Foundation, Fred Mann and David Morse (prior to his leaving) offered wise counsel to the editors. After Morse's departure, Mann played a critical role in shaping this volume, and we are especially grateful to him. In addition to reading every chapter, Risa Lavizzo-Mourey provided guidance and support. Molly McKaughan reviewed the entire volume for accuracy and consistency. Rose Littman, Tina Hines, and Melissa Blair facilitated communication between the San Francisco–based editor and the Foundation's staff and made it seem easy. Mimi Turi continued her outstanding work on contractual and administrative matters with Health Policy Associates. Mary Castria, Carol Owle, Carolyn Scholer, and Chris Sowa handled financial matters efficiently. Mary Beth Kren located, as she has done in the past, materials that otherwise would have been impossible to obtain. Andrew Harrison organized the Foundation's oral history and guided the editors through it.

Hope Woodhead, Joan Barlow, and Sherry DeMarchi handled distribution deftly. Ed Ghisu negotiated the contract with Jossey-Bass. Patti Higgins, assisted by Tejal Shah, reviewed the final drafts of the manuscript and made the editors feel comfortable that all references to Foundation programs were accurate; she did additional, and much appreciated, copyediting. Penny Bolla and the web team worked with the editors to make sure that material in the book appeared promptly and accurately on the Foundation's website.

At Jossey-Bass, Andy Pasternack, Seth Schwartz, and Justin Frahm did a highly professional job in producing the *Anthology*.

We would like to recognize the outstanding contribution made by Amy Woodrum, the research and evaluation assistant at the Foundation. Amy was a full partner in putting together this volume of the *Anthology*, and we are greatly appreciative of the high quality of her work.

Finally, to those who shaped the stories covered throughout this volume, we owe a debt of gratitude for embodying the values and spirit of the Robert Wood Johnson Foundation.

S.L.I. and D.C.C.

Section One

The Robert Wood Johnson Foundation at Forty

—∿— Editors' Introduction to Section One

This first section of Volume XV offers readers an overview of the Robert Wood Johnson Foundation and its evolution over the past forty years. It begins with two original chapters, which are followed by reprints of *Anthology* chapters that illuminate specific aspects of the Foundation.

The section begins with a brief history of the Foundation, written by the editors and Sarah G. Pickell, who was a research assistant at the Foundation when the chapter was drafted and is currently the director of communications and development at the University of Virginia's Institute for Advanced Studies in Culture. In conducting their research for the chapter, the authors were granted access to many interviews with the Foundation's leaders, including its founders, conducted by Joel Gardner between 1991 and 2011 for the Foundation's oral history. This is the first time that excerpts from the materials in the oral history files, which previously had been off limits, are being made publicly available.

The chapter takes us from the period when Robert Wood Johnson established the Foundation's predecessor, called the Johnson New Brunswick Foundation, through the current Foundation's establishment as a national philanthropy in 1972 and up to the present day. It looks at the Foundation through the administrations of each of its presidents: David Rogers (1972–1986), Leighton Cluff (1986–1990), Steven Schroeder (1990–2002), and Risa Lavizzo-Mourey (2003–present). Since Lavizzo-Mourey's presidency is still ongoing and doesn't afford the same possibility for a retrospective look that the three earlier presidencies do, the section on her administration is, by necessity, considerably briefer than the preceding ones.

That brevity is more than compensated for by Chapter 2, a conversation with Lavizzo-Mourey as she completes her tenth year as the Foundation's president and CEO. The conversation distills four separate hour-long interviews conducted by Stephen Isaacs. In this chapter, Lavizzo-Mourey—who holds both medical and business degrees and, prior to coming to the Foundation, had been a gerontologist, a Robert Wood Johnson Clinical Scholar, a medical school professor, a clinician, a researcher, and a government official—offers a rare look into her background and the influences on her career and shares her thoughts on the Foundation, its work to date, and the challenges ahead.

These two original chapters are followed by reprints of six chapters that appeared in earlier volumes of the *Anthology*. The first of the reprints examines the life, philosophy, and legacy of the legendary Foundation official Terry Keenan. The next five examine a particular element of the Foundation's work—philanthropic approaches employed by the Foundation (the five Cs), evaluation, communications, national programs, and New Jersey programs. Each reprint is preceded by an editors' introduction that places it in context and brings it up to date.

CHAPTER 1

The Robert Wood Johnson Foundation at Forty

David C. Colby, Stephen L. Isaacs, and Sarah G. Pickell

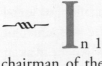In 1936, Robert Wood Johnson, the president and chairman of the board of Johnson & Johnson, established the Johnson New Brunswick Foundation to conduct his charitable giving in New Brunswick and Middlesex Counties, New Jersey. For the first three and a half decades of its existence, the foundation—which in 1952 became the Robert Wood Johnson Foundation—made nearly all of its donations to hospitals and other health care organizations, community-service programs, nursing, scholarships, and aid to the indigent.

Robert Wood Johnson died in 1968. After providing for family members, he left the bulk of his estate—shares in Johnson & Johnson (J&J)—to the foundation bearing his name. By the time the estate was settled three years later, the shares were valued at $1.2 billion, making the Robert Wood Johnson Foundation the second richest foundation in the nation. In fact, the night after the new Foundation's endowment was reported in the newspapers, burglars broke into the Foundation's offices on Livingston Avenue in New Brunswick looking to help themselves to the $1.2 billion. They left empty-handed.

The Foundation's early trustees were, for the most part, current and past senior executives at J&J (a notable exception being William McChesney Martin, a former chairman of the Federal Reserve Board). Gustav Lienhard, the former J&J chief financial officer and chairman of the company's executive committee, chaired the Foundation Board with an iron hand until his retirement in 1985. Early on, the Board determined that in accordance with Robert Wood Johnson's interests, the new philanthropy would concentrate on advancing health and health care in the United States, and to press that agenda, it recruited David Rogers, the dean of the Johns Hopkins Medical School, as the Foundation's first president.

—⁓— The David Rogers Era: 1972–1986

A physician, teacher, and researcher, Rogers had challenged racial discrimination at Vanderbilt University when he was chief of medicine there, served the poor of Baltimore when he was at Johns Hopkins, and supported the passage of Medicare and Medicaid. "I came up to meet with the Board, and had a meeting with all or most of the trustees in the J&J headquarters," Rogers recalled in an interview. "After fifteen or twenty minutes, I realized this group was on a totally different, very conservative, wavelength. 'The thing that puzzles me,' I said, 'is why me? We disagree on virtually every social issue. You know, among my friends, I'm considered a liberal.' Philip Hofmann, who was then the J&J chairman and was on the Foundation Board, turned to me and said, 'We don't care what your politics are. We aim to make this the best foundation in the world, and we think you can do that.' And I thought, 'Okay, why not give it a try!'"[1]

Rogers quickly brought on a first-rate staff, many of whom would go on to have stellar careers in their own right: for example, Margaret Mahoney would head The Commonwealth Fund; Robert Blendon would become a leading health care survey researcher at Harvard University; Linda Aiken (whom Rogers recruited in 1974) would become a prominent nursing researcher and leader; Terrance Keenan would become a legendary grantmaker at the Robert Wood Johnson Foundation. As his special adviser, Rogers recruited Walsh McDermott, who had already won an Albert Lasker Award for his medical research. His role at the Foundation involved coaching Rogers and his staff, as well as providing counsel.

Rogers and his team established principles for the Foundation that still resonate forty years later. They agreed that the Foundation's grantmaking should be targeted—focusing on only a few selected areas of major concern. "We were going to be a rifle, not a shotgun," Rogers said. They also decided to focus the Foundation's grantmaking on what Blendon called "investment activities," that is, grants that would have a long-term payoff, as compared to short-term charitable grants.[2]

The idea of national programs developed early in the Rogers administration. With the guidance of experts in each particular area, the Foundation would design a program and outsource the selection of grantees, administration, and monitoring to a partner organization, usually headed by a leader in the field. If all went well, the federal government would pick up the funding of the program. As a side benefit, these national programs would also attract a network of influential people committed to the same goals. "What we did was get people involved who were a *Who's Who* in American health care," Blendon recalled. "We got them very interested in the programs, and they became much more important advocates for changes and innovations than we could be." By 1975, there were eight national programs.

To measure results, the Foundation commissioned outside researchers to assess large projects where the potential for measuring outcomes was great, and it hired an evaluation staff to oversee this work. To disseminate results, Rogers recruited a communications staff and named Frank Karel as the Foundation's first vice president of communications, fulfilling Rogers's vision of "a top senior officer concerned with public affairs who will participate fully in the discussion of policy, the selection of areas of focus, and the considerations of proposals we plan to support."[3] In this role, Karel pioneered the concept of strategic communications in philanthropy.

Programming: 1972–1980

The Foundation's initial challenge was to comply with the federal requirement to spend a percentage of its net assets amounting to roughly $45 million the first year. "We picked some big programs we thought couldn't go wrong," Rogers said. "We put a big chunk into needy students in medicine, and bent it quite sharply toward minority students. We did several things like that, which didn't require a lot of research on the part of the Foundation."

Rogers and the staff then turned to the more substantial challenge of determining longer-term priorities. They sought the guidance of experts, holding a two-day meeting in March 1972 with leaders from medicine, economics, law, and government to discuss objectives for the new foundation. Then Rogers and Foundation vice president Blendon set to work mapping out a course of action. "David and I agreed pretty quickly that it was important to find a niche," Blendon recalled. "Access to care was what Rogers had been about. Then we added quality and public policy." In May 1972, Rogers presented the Board with the Foundation's three priorities—increasing access to medical services, improving the quality of care, and providing objective information on health care policy. The Board voted its approval.

Access to Care

"Although some segments of society had been particularly inadequately served, *no* group of that day was without problems in obtaining fully satisfactory, easily accessible health care...

especially for those who were ill but not in need of hospitalization," Blendon, Aiken, and Rogers recalled.[4] The challenge, they argued, was in providing "health services of the right kind at the right time to the right person." To do this, the Foundation employed three strategies.

To serve the millions of people expected to be covered under the health reform proposed, but never enacted, during the Nixon Administration, the first strategy sought to expand the number and types of health professionals. The Foundation supported the training of medical students and residents committed to primary care and to serving in inner-city and rural areas. "Being the major foundation in health that was supporting primary care, we made generalist physicians kind of legitimate," Rogers remembered. "At the time, everything was going in the other direction—to the subspecialties."

But the Foundation did not rely solely on physicians to provide care; it launched programs to train nurse practitioners and physician assistants, at a time when both professions were in their infancy. The Foundation even funded a program to train health aides in Alaska to care for their neighbors in isolated rural communities. The dental profession was included as well, through both scholarships and training opportunities.

The second strategy was to demonstrate new approaches to providing health care services, with an eye cocked toward the federal government. "David Rogers and I always understood that the federal government was the buyer," Blendon said. The nation's hospitals were a logical place to start, and the Foundation quickly embarked on initiatives to encourage hospitals of all stripes (community, municipal, and teaching hospitals) to beef up their ambulatory care services.

Although the hospital programs were the main focus of the Foundation's efforts to increase access to ambulatory care, probably the best known of the early demonstration programs is the one that helped create an emergency medical system. After the Department of Health, Education, and Welfare funded five emergency medical services demonstration projects in 1972, the Robert Wood Johnson Foundation provided $15 million to expand the concept to forty-four additional sites. Ultimately, the federal government picked up funding of emergency medical services, and the idea—which we now know as the 9–1–1 emergency phone number—spread throughout the country.

During this period, the Foundation also launched the School Health Services Program in four elementary schools, where nurse practitioners treated the students. Thus began the Foundation's long support of school-based health services, which expanded over the years, continuing through the early 2000s. It became, however, a controversial area. "Many people were pushing back," former Foundation vice president Peter Goodwin recalls. "The Foundation was seen as dispensing birth control in high schools. But it was really about basic primary care in schools."[5] School health services are now available in approximately two thousand schools in forty-four states.

The third strategy the Foundation used to increase access to care was supporting research. In 1974, for example, the Foundation funded Ronald Andersen and Lu Ann Aday of the University of Chicago to conduct the first in a series of influential access-to-care surveys. "The access-to-care studies gave us a lot of legitimacy in the health policy community as a national research-based foundation," former Foundation vice president Aiken said. "It established the Foundation as a serious player."[6] The Foundation also supported an important study by Robert Mendenhall and his colleagues at the University of Southern California School of Medicine which found that specialists were providing more primary care than had previously been thought.

Quality of Care

The second goal of this period was improving quality of health care, including prevention of illness by means such as better nutrition and more physical activity. Forty years later, in the context of the childhood obesity epidemic, nutrition and physical activity have become even more important. Presciently, in 1972, the Foundation gave a grant to physician-researcher Lawrence Weed of the University of Vermont to support his work developing an early version of an electronic medical record.

Additionally, the Foundation adopted the Clinical Scholars program, which had been started by The Commonwealth Fund and the Carnegie Corporation of New York, and expanded it substantially. Under this program, physicians would study epidemiology or the social sciences in order to gain the breadth of knowledge needed to become leaders in the field. Among the more than 1,100 alumni of this signature Foundation program, which the health policy experts Rashi Fein and John Rowe termed "a national treasure," are many of the nation's most influential leaders in health services and health policy.

The Clinical Scholars Program provided the model for a program, launched in 1982, to develop leaders of the nursing profession. "The idea behind the Clinical Nurse Scholars Program," said Aiken, "was to take people who already had their education and, through a postdoctoral experience, retool them in research and clinical care. The only way that nurses could get stature and authority in university settings was to be expert researchers." Many of its sixty two graduates went on to become leaders of the nursing profession.

Public Policy

The third goal was to improve the way health policy was formulated. To reach it, the Foundation helped build organizations— most notably the National Health Policy Forum at The George Washington University and the Institute for Health Policy Studies (now the Philip R. Lee Institute for Health Policy Studies) at the University of California, San Francisco—to provide high-quality information to policymakers.

With an eye toward developing the field of health services research, the Foundation supported researchers, many of whom, such as Karen Davis, Paul Ginsburg, Harold Luft, and William Hsiao, have become prominent in the field. It also created the Health Policy Fellows program, which gave, and continues to give, midcareer health professionals from academic centers the opportunity to work in a congressional or federal government office. This program has graduated more than two hundred fellows.

One little known program that had an important influence on public policy was the National Hospice Study. Launched in 1980 in collaboration with the federal government and the John A. Hartford Foundation, the study took place in the midst of a national debate on the treatment of terminally ill patients. The preliminary results were used to design a new Medicare hospice benefit that began in 1982. According to Aiken, the study "created a groundswell political movement that got the whole hospice movement off the ground."

Programming: 1981–1986

Beginning in 1977, the Foundation began reviewing its priorities in light of the changing health care landscape. National health insurance had not materialized, and Robert Mendenhall's research had revealed that although access to care remained a serious problem, the situation was better than had been previously thought. However, "the financing system in America was getting worse," Blendon recalled. "More people were uninsured. The government was not funding inner-city programs . . . we were in a situation where, rather than being ahead of the wave, we were out there by ourselves."

The review led the Foundation's leadership, in 1980, to refocus its work. It established three priorities: First, it would continue its work to improve access to health services, but focus that work on the underserved. Second, in an attempt to address the issue of rising medical costs, it would strive to make health care more effective and affordable. Third, it would aim to improve services for people with chronic conditions. In addition, the Foundation agreed to commit funds to improve diversity in the health professions.

Access to Care

Between 1981 and 1986, the Foundation allocated about a third of its grant dollars to improving access for particularly vulnerable populations. These included homeless people. The Health Care for the Homeless Program, funded in collaboration with The Pew Charitable Trusts, provided health and social services to homeless people in eighteen states and became the model for the federal McKinney Homeless Assistance Act of 1987.

Children born into difficult circumstances comprised another vulnerable population. Largely under the leadership of Ruby Hearn, at the time a Foundation program officer (she later became a vice president and then the senior vice president), the Foundation launched many programs aimed at improving children's health. These included programs to send registered nurses into the homes of poor pregnant single women to teach them how to care for themselves during their pregnancy and how to care for their children after they are born,[7] to develop networks of perinatal care hospitals in rural areas,[8] and to continue bringing health care into the nation's elementary and secondary schools.[9]

Effectiveness and Affordability

In the early 1980s, the rising cost of health care emerged as an important concern, and the Foundation responded by funding a variety of demonstration programs and research projects testing different ways of reining in costs. The Foundation's primary effort was the Community Programs for Affordable Health Care, to determine whether community-based groups could contain health care costs. An evaluation found that the effort did not succeed because communities simply did not have the power to lower the cost of health care. None of the Foundation-funded programs succeeded in finding lasting ways to reduce costs, and this priority was soon abandoned.

Chronic Conditions

In his 1981 president's message, David Rogers noted that more than thirty million Americans had "health-related functional limitations that interfere with their effectiveness." That same year, the Foundation funded several programs to address issues of chronic illness. Perhaps the most successful, in terms of results and longevity, was On Lok, a San Francisco-based program that provided integrated acute and long-term care for low-income, nursing-home-eligible seniors, enabling them to remain in their homes. With the inclusion of the Program for All-Inclusive Care for the Elderly in the Balanced Budget Act of 1997, the federal government adopted the On Lok approach as one available for people eligible for both Medicare and Medicaid. State governments, however, have been cautious in adopting the approach.

By 1986, AIDS had become the nation's most visible health problem. "It was very controversial within the Foundation," says the former Foundation vice president Paul Jellinek. "Even so, it was too important for the nation's largest health foundation to ignore. So David Rogers asked Drew Altman, who was then a Foundation vice president, and me to go to San Francisco and check out an apparently effective program that was providing care in the community to people with AIDS." Subsequently, the Foundation authorized the AIDS Health Services Program to replicate the San Francisco approach in eleven other cities. When Congress passed the Ryan White Act (the vehicle through which federal AIDS prevention and treatment programs are funded) in 1990, it adopted the Foundation's community-based approach.

In recognition of the Foundation's work, Rogers was named the vice chairman of the National Commission on AIDS after his retirement from the Foundation.

Diversity

In addition to the fellowship programs begun earlier in the Rogers era to train physicians, nurses, and dentists, the Foundation sought to attract minorities to the health professions and to bolster their chances of succeeding. In 1983, the Foundation began the Minority Medical Faculty Development Program (now named after Harold Amos, the first African American to chair a department at the Harvard Medical School) to increase the number of minority faculty members at nonminority medical schools, even as it supported faculty development at the nation's historically black medical colleges. The commitment to minorities in the health field has characterized the Foundation ever since.

Looking Back at the Rogers Years

"It was Rogers' vision that made the Foundation," Aiken said. "He had a notion that the Foundation was going to be like a quasi-university ... a place where intellectuals, but intellectuals who knew how to do something, would come together and take advantage of the incredible opportunity of having money to test ideas." In the Rogers era, the DNA of the Robert Wood Johnson Foundation was created. In program terms, it can be simply stated: research a problem; build a national program to address it; evaluate the solutions; and communicate the results in the hopes that the federal government would adopt and finance the idea. In other words, at a time when government was viewed positively, the Foundation saw its role as the research and development arm of the health care field. In some cases, such as health care for homeless people, AIDS services, and the On Lok model of community care for seniors, the government did pick up programs piloted by the Foundation. In other cases, such as nurse practitioners and physician assistants, the fields became part of the mainstream, facilitated by market forces and government support.

Part of the Foundation's DNA had to do with developing leaders through programs such as Clinical Scholars and providing the opportunity for minorities to become health professionals, another enduring commitment. Still another legacy from those years is the Foundation's emphasis on research, evaluation, and communications. Perhaps most significant, during the Rogers era, the Foundation became strategic and mission-driven—addressing long-term solutions for a limited number of health care issues affecting the most vulnerable segments of American society.

—⌇— The Leighton Cluff Era: 1986–1990

When David Rogers retired in 1986, the Board, now chaired by attorney Robert Myers, named as his successor Leighton Cluff, who had chaired the Department of Medicine at the University of Florida before becoming the Foundation's executive vice president in 1976. Both Cluff and Myers viewed themselves as short-term appointments. "I had not intended to be the president very long because I wanted to retire," Cluff said. "It had become clear to me that Bob Myers also looked upon himself as a person who was not going to stay very long."[10]

For Cluff, the health care environment required the Foundation to become more flexible and responsive. He was willing to let a thousand flowers bloom in the hope of growing one that was gorgeous. The saying, "Before you find a prince you have to kiss a lot of frogs," was framed on his office wall. Moreover, the Foundation staff "was beginning to recognize that many of the health problems they needed to address were inextricably intertwined with social problems," according to Alan Cohen, the vice president for research and evaluation under Cluff.[11] This, too, was a change from the Rogers era, when health care was the predominant, almost singular, focus.

Cluff significantly broadened the way that communications were used. During his tenure, the Foundation gave its first grant to support news coverage—to WGBH in 1988 for *The AIDS Quarterly*, hosted by news anchor Peter Jennings. The award-winning program was later expanded into *The Health Quarterly*. The Foundation, also for the first time, funded a targeted public relations effort by supporting, beginning in 1989, the media campaigns of the Partnership for a Drug-Free America.

Although Cluff strongly supported evaluation, Cohen changed the focus somewhat, emphasizing formative evaluation because, he said, "It was important to us to feed information back that could strengthen the program."

Although Cluff had been considered a disciple of Rogers, under his administration programming took a different turn. He wanted to open up the Foundation to new areas and new—mainly community-based—grantees. In keeping with this philosophy, Cluff broadened the Foundation's grantmaking priorities from three to ten.[12] Interestingly, the priorities did not include access to care. "That traditional focus of Foundation support was diminished, in order to direct energies and resources on those populations most likely to be overlooked in a generally improved (albeit still imperfect) health care delivery system," Cluff said.[13] As expected under this approach to grantmaking, some areas were effective and long-lived while many fell by the wayside. The following are among the highlights of the Cluff era's programs.

Research into the Organization, Financing, and Delivery of Health Care Services

Through the Changes in Health Care Financing and Organization (HCFO) initiative, the Foundation helped strengthen the field of health services research, nurtured many of the field's leading researchers, and provided information upon which policies could be based. The initiative remains active today. The Foundation also funded research into many of the pressing issues of the time.

For example, a major study that looked at medical malpractice reached conclusions that continue to be cited today, and the largely negative findings from the Health Care for the Uninsured Program, designed to find ways for small employers to insure their employees, remain pertinent.

Mental Health

In the mid-1980s, the Foundation launched two programs to improve the disorganized systems of delivering mental health services. The first, the Program on Chronic Mental Illness, which was carried out in collaboration with the U.S. Department of Housing and Urban Development in nine cities, sought to centralize responsibility for mental health services in a single agency. The second, the Mental Health Services Program for Youth, encouraged state and local partnerships to coordinate care for children with mental health problems; the $19 million provided by the Foundation was the largest single influx of money into the children's mental health system up to that time. Both programs provided models for better coordination of mental health services and underscored the importance of improving the quality of mental health services, in addition to the systems by which they are delivered.

Long-Term Care

In the late 1980s, the issue of older people impoverishing themselves in order to qualify for Medicaid coverage of nursing-home care received national attention. To address this issue, the Foundation developed, in 1987, a program to test a new way of financing long-term care. Under the Program to Promote Long-Term Care Insurance for the Elderly, private insurance companies and governments of four states entered into partnerships whereby seniors who purchased private long-term care insurance policies would not have to spend down their resources to receive Medicaid.

Although the results were disappointing (people bought far fewer policies than the originators had expected, and buyers tended to have higher incomes than had been envisioned), the model proved attractive to Congress which, in the Deficit Reduction Act of 2005, allowed Medicaid programs in all states to adopt long-term care insurance partnerships.

To allow people with dementia to live at home, the Foundation funded two programs that examined the potential of adult day-care centers.[14] These programs showed that such centers could effectively serve people with chronic illness and provide respite to caregivers.

AIDS

Cluff continued the Foundation's work to combat AIDS that had begun toward the end of the Rogers era, but expanded the approach to prevention—not just treatment—of the disease. The AIDS Prevention and Services Project sought to attract a broad set of community-based grantees by simplifying the application process, providing a telephone hotline to help applicants, and asking potential applicants for proposals that would organize prevention services as they saw appropriate. "It was an unprecedented undertaking for the Foundation to do both an open-ended call for proposals and for it to be on AIDS," recalled the former senior vice president Ruby Hearn. "More than one thousand organizations applied—many of them community groups. This was an overwhelming response."

Substance Abuse

In the late 1980s, the nation found itself in the throes of a drug epidemic that many people felt threatened the very fabric of society. The Foundation developed a three-pronged approach to addressing it. The first prong was a program called Fighting Back, which started in 1988 and continued until 2003. It was an $88 million program to assist community-led coalitions to implement a variety of anti-drug and anti-alcohol abuse strategies. Shortly after it began, the federal government adopted the model and expanded it to 251 sites. The second prong, a companion program, Join Together, which remains active today even after Foundation funding has ended, provided technical assistance to community coalitions and information for the field and for policymakers. The third prong, Community Anti-Drug Coalitions of America, addressed, and continues to address, policy issues directly on behalf of its community-coalition members.

End-of-Life Care

Toward the end of Cluff's tenure, the Foundation launched a major research study into the care given to hospitalized, terminally ill patients. The findings from the Study to Understand Prognoses and Preferences for Outcomes and Risks of Treatments, or SUPPORT as it was called, did not become available until 1995. When the negative results were released, they led the Foundation to embark on a widely praised effort to reform the care of dying patients.

Looking Back at the Cluff Years

Because the Cluff era was a relatively short, transitional one, it is difficult to judge whether his approach to philanthropy— experimenting with many different priorities and approaches in the hopes of finding some that work—would have succeeded. Moreover, it was a political period—the Reagan-Bush years—when the federal government was less likely to pick up successful programs than it had been under previous administrations. Perhaps the most noteworthy feature of the Cluff era was its recognition that people's health depended on more than increased access to medical services—that it depended on social and behavioral considerations as well. As the Foundation's oral historian, Joel Gardner, observed, "By making substance abuse a priority,

Cluff set the stage for the Foundation's later work to combat smoking. And his efforts to engage the issue of AIDS, along with social and behavioral health problems, presaged the Foundation's later reorganization into health and health care components."[15] Finally, the Foundation's use of communications as an intervention itself, through the *AIDS Quarterly* television show, led to an expansion of the Foundation's approach to communications in later years.

The Steven Schroeder Era: 1990–2002

Sidney Wentz, the former chairman and CEO of the insurance company Crum & Forster, replaced Robert Myers as the Foundation's Board chairman in 1989. The following year, the Board named Steven Schroeder, a general internist and professor at the University of California, San Francisco, as the Foundation's third president.

Schroeder quickly sharpened the Foundation's focus to three strategic priorities: expanding access to care, improving chronic illness care, and reducing the harm caused by substance abuse, especially smoking. He presented this agenda to the Board at a retreat in February 1991. "Most of the debate focused on substance abuse and whether or not cigarettes and alcohol should be in," Schroeder recalled. "The debate got very heated."[16] Board members worried that the reputation of the Robert Wood Johnson Foundation would be sullied by getting into conflict with the tobacco companies. "Ultimately, we had a vote whether we should go with substance abuse, and it was eight to eight. At that point, we evolved a compromise that we would keep alcohol and tobacco in but focus on youth only."

Containing the cost of medical care emerged as a mini-priority but was quickly abandoned as beyond the reach of the Foundation to influence, just as it had been abandoned earlier.

The extraordinary growth of the Foundation's endowment during the boom years of the 1990s (assets tripled from roughly

$3 billion in 1990 to nearly $9 billion in 1998) stimulated a discussion of how the money should be spent and how the Foundation should be organized. Initially, Schroeder proposed using some of the endowment to establish a separate foundation concentrating only on substance abuse. The Board nixed that idea. But in 1997, it approved a reorganization of the Foundation into two groups: one devoted to health care (headed initially by Jack Ebeler and, after April 2001, by Risa Lavizzo-Mourey) and the other to health (headed by J. Michael McGinnis). "I wanted to see if we could institutionalize the health part," Schroeder said.

During Schroeder's tenure, communications—led by Frank Karel and, upon his retirement at the end of 2001, by David Morse—became increasingly used as a strategic tool, as seen by the annual Cover the Uninsured Week, the advocacy work of the Center for Tobacco-Free Kids, and the coalition building of the Last Acts program. With the recruitment of a new vice president, James Knickman, the Foundation made evaluation more relevant to program staff and conducted research into areas of interest to policymakers. It measured performance toward reaching its program goals quantitatively and through an annual "scorecard" that measured not just results for program areas but also for the Foundation's own management performance and reputation in the field. The communications and research and evaluation units collaborated in developing Grant Results Reports, now known as Program Results Reports, and the *Anthology* series to examine programs and clusters of programs, and to share the findings widely.

Although it is difficult to prove the value of fellowship programs quantitatively, Schroeder—and his two executive vice presidents, Richard Reynolds through 1996 and Lewis Sandy between 1997 and 2002—believed in their value. Not only did Schroeder expand the Foundation's ongoing Clinical Scholars and Health Policy Fellows programs, he also added new ones to strengthen research and to attract more minorities to the health professions. Schroeder also revitalized the Local Initiative Funding Partners Program (now known as the Robert Wood Johnson

Foundation Local Funding Partnerships program), under which the Foundation collaborated with local foundations to expand promising community-level programs.

Programmatically, the Schroeder era is perhaps best characterized by the Foundation's programs to reduce smoking (and, to a lesser extent, substance abuse), improve end-of-life care, expand health insurance coverage, improve chronic care, and advance primary care.

Tobacco Control

Between 1991 and 2002, under the leadership of Schroeder and Nancy Kaufman, whom Schroeder brought on as a vice president to oversee the Foundation's tobacco control and other substance abuse programs, the Foundation invested more than $700 million in a wide-ranging effort to reduce tobacco use. As it evolved over the decade, the Foundation's approach contained four elements: research, advocacy and policy, coalition building, and smoking cessation.

Research

Through its Tobacco Policy Research and Evaluation Program and its successor, the Substance Abuse Policy Research Program, the Foundation created a field of tobacco-policy research whose findings influenced policy throughout the country. Frank Chaloupka at the University of Illinois at Chicago, for example, documented that increasing the tax on a pack of cigarettes would reduce sales—especially to young people—and provided the rationale for increasing excise taxes on cigarettes. John Slade, a professor at the University of Medicine & Dentistry of New Jersey, analyzed the tobacco industry and public documents, leading to a better understanding of the addictive nature of nicotine—which in turn provided the underpinning for the U.S. Food and Drug Administration's being given authority to regulate tobacco products in 2009.

Advocacy and Policy

In 1996, the Foundation established the National Center for Tobacco-Free Kids (now known as the Campaign for Tobacco-Free Kids) to serve as the voice of tobacco control and a counterweight to the tobacco industry. The center quickly established a national network of thousands of grassroots advocates, spokespersons, and alliances dedicated to reducing children's tobacco use. Nationally, it played a leading role in negotiating a settlement of a lawsuit brought by state attorneys general to require the major tobacco companies to reimburse state governments for Medicaid costs expended on persons treated for tobacco-related diseases.

Coalition Building

The third element in the Foundation's strategy—organizing and financing local and state coalitions to be advocates for tobacco-control policies—fell primarily to the American Medical Association in its role as the national program office for the SmokeLess States Program. From 1993 to 2004, the work of SmokeLess States coalitions contributed to increased tobacco taxes in thirty-five states, clean indoor-air legislation in ten states, and ordinances to restrict young people's access to tobacco products in thirteen states.[17]

Helping Smokers Quit

The Foundation's staff and its grantees sought to translate research findings into practical smoking-cessation guidelines (such guidelines were adopted by both the U.S. Public Health Service and the National Committee for Quality Assurance) and programs that could be adopted by employers and covered by insurance.

In 2011, the Foundation released an independent analysis of its tobacco-control work. Even recognizing the difficulty of attributing behavioral change on a national level to any single player, the analysis concluded that "The Robert Wood Johnson Foundation's contributions were significant."[18]

Alcohol and Illicit Drugs

At a time when few foundations were interested in alcohol and illicit substance addiction, the Robert Wood Johnson Foundation made combatting it a priority and funded both research studies and demonstration projects. The College Alcohol Studies, a series of surveys on drinking by college students, conducted by the Harvard University researcher Henry Wechsler between 1992 and 2006, alerted the nation to binge drinking on the nation's campuses. Research conducted under the auspices of the Substance Abuse Policy Research Program revealed, among other things, that office-based methadone treatment was effective and that lives can be saved by automobile ignition devices that prevent a car from starting if a driver is drunk. Research by the National Center on Addiction and Substance Abuse, and its promotion by the center's president, former Health, Education, and Welfare Secretary Joseph Califano, received considerable media coverage and heightened awareness of the extent and consequences of substance abuse. The Bridging the Gap program became a major source of data on adolescent smoking, drinking, and illicit drug use.

Demonstration programs were mounted to test the effectiveness of community anti-substance-abuse coalitions;[19] to support community development efforts through community coalitions working with local Head Start organizations;[20] and to improve systems of treating young people with substance-abuse addictions who are in the juvenile justice system.[21] Spurred by the College Alcohol Studies, the Foundation developed programs to reduce binge drinking on college campuses[22] and to prevent the sale of alcohol to high school students.[23]

By the late 1990s, new knowledge—especially about the neurobiology of addiction—had demonstrated the possibility of treating addiction with medication. But there was still little financing for treatment, and the available care was often not only of low quality but was delivered in a fragmented system. In the last year of the Schroeder era, 2002, the Foundation funded two new programs aimed at improving access to, and the quality of, addiction treatment.[24]

To build public awareness, the Foundation sponsored, in 1998, a five-part PBS television series on addiction and recovery, hosted by Bill Moyers. It also funded the Entertainment Industries Council's PRISM Awards to those in the entertainment industry who most accurately depicted tobacco, alcohol, and drug abuse.

An assessment of the Foundation's drug abuse programs published in Volume XIII of the *Anthology* concluded, "On balance, the Foundation's sizable investment in addiction prevention and treatment was considered a qualified success, weakened by a lack of a strong, steady strategic vision, episodic program decisions, and some institutional infighting. And looming constantly over the fragmented drug addiction work was the Foundation's signature accomplishment: its highly regarded efforts to reduce smoking. It proved to be a very tough act to follow."[25]

End-of-Life/Palliative Care

When the results of SUPPORT, the large research study designed to test ways to improve the care of dying patients, were released in 1995, they were devastating. Despite specially trained nurses who counseled terminally ill hospitalized patients and their families about their options, patients were still not receiving the kind of care they wanted and, contrary to their wishes, were tethered to machines. In response to this discouraging news, the Foundation developed a multiyear, multicomponent initiative to improve the care of dying patients.

The first component was to increase the knowledge and capacity of health care professionals in caring for dying patients. The Foundation funded the development of training programs for physicians and nurses, encouraged publishers to incorporate material on end-of-life care in medical and nursing textbooks, and supported a regular series in the *Journal of the American Medical Association* to bring end-of-life care to the attention of physicians.

The second component was to improve palliative care[26] in hospitals and other health care institutions. To this end, with support from the Foundation, the Center to Advance Palliative Care at New York City's Mount Sinai Medical Center became a national resource for research, information, technical assistance, and training on palliative care. Palliative care has grown rapidly. It is now offered in most major hospitals and is recognized as a subspecialty by the American Board of Medical Specialties.

The third component was to modify state regulations on pain management so that physicians could prescribe, without fear of prosecution, controlled substances to patients suffering great pain. Thanks in part to Foundation-funded work by the University of Wisconsin School of Medicine and Public Health—which provided information and assistance to state attorneys general and other government officials—thirty-five states modified their pain-management policies between 2000 and 2007.

The Foundation supplemented these efforts with an aggressive outreach and communications effort that developed community coalitions through the Last Acts program; publications, such as the *Five Wishes* booklet, that publicized living wills, health care proxies, and durable powers of attorney; and a four-part PBS series on death and dying in America, *On Our Own Terms*, hosted by Bill Moyers, which was watched by more viewers than any other program in U.S. public television history up to that time.

An independent retrospective analysis of the Foundation's end-of-life programs concluded, "The achievements are remarkable . . . the impact is being felt in the actual practice of medicine."[27]

Access to Care

Given Schroeder's earlier work to promote primary care, it is not surprising that soon after his arrival the Foundation launched a series of programs to increase the supply of generalist physicians—general internists, general pediatricians, and family practitioners.[28] For a brief period in the mid-1990s—when it appeared that primary care would take off under managed care—academic medicine appeared receptive to generalist medicine. But as managed-care expansion slowed in the late-1990s following a consumer backlash, medical schools reverted to their historical preferences for specialists and basic research.

While the generalist physician programs concentrated on increasing the *supply* of primary-care doctors, other programs focused on their *distribution* and included health professionals other than doctors. The Foundation employed a variety of approaches: testing different ways to recruit primary-care providers to underserved areas;[29] encouraging physicians to volunteer their services to uninsured people;[30] using distance-learning techniques to train nurse practitioners, nurse-midwives, and physician assistants in their own homes, often in rural areas;[31] and offering incentives to attract health professionals to work in the rural South, where people had less access to care than anywhere else in the nation.[32]

When President Clinton announced, in early 1993, the establishment of a task force to develop a plan to provide health insurance coverage for all Americans, the Foundation, which had long been waiting for such a moment, turned its attention to health reform. It made the considerable body of Foundation-funded research on health insurance and coverage easily available to policymakers. More visibly, it organized four *Conversations on Health*—widely publicized meetings designed to raise public awareness about the importance of expanding insurance coverage. Schroeder chaired three of the four meetings. "We made a very serious effort to keep the forums evenhanded, inviting

Republicans as well as Democrats to attend," former Board chairman Wentz recalled. "But it turned out that mostly Democrats attended."[33] The Foundation received withering Republican criticism for engaging in partisan politics. In retrospect, according to Brown University political scientist James Morone, the Foundation appears to have unwittingly gotten caught in the crossfire of internal Republican politics.[34]

After the defeat of the Clinton health-reform plan and stung by the accusations of partisanship, the Foundation turned its attention to the states while simultaneously monitoring the changes taking place in the health care system and trying to keep the idea of national health reform alive.

At the state and local levels, the Foundation funded experiments to expand health insurance coverage,[35] giving particular attention to insuring children. Through its Covering Kids & Families Initiative, the Foundation gave states support in conducting outreach, simplifying the enrollment and renewal processes, and coordinating enrollment of children eligible for Medicaid or the State Children's Health Insurance Program. The initiative was supplemented by a large-scale communications effort built around annual Back to School campaigns, which grassroots activists used to enroll needy kids in health insurance programs. Between 1997 and 2002, a time when the number of uninsured adults was rising, the number of uninsured children dropped from 11 to 8 million.

To monitor the changes occurring in health care, especially the rise of managed care, the Foundation created the Center for Studying Health System Change in 1995. The Center, which now receives support from many sources, has become an influential source of information for government policymakers. The Foundation also continued funding research on health insurance and access to care by the Urban Institute and the Economic Research Initiative on the Uninsured at the University of Michigan.

To keep the issue of health insurance coverage alive, even after it had dropped off the national policy agenda with the failure of health reform in 1994, the Foundation funded six reports by the Institute of Medicine between 2000 and 2004 on the uninsured and the consequences of being without health insurance. The reports generated widespread national attention, as did the Foundation-funded "strange bedfellows" group. The group brought together an unlikely coalition of labor, business, insurers, hospitals, nurses, physicians, and consumer advocates to see if they could find common ground. In fact, they were able to do so, and in 2000 the group issued a statement highlighting that most of the uninsured were working Americans and that the consequences of not being insured could be devastating. The work of the strange bedfellows led to the Cover the Uninsured Week campaigns between 2003 and 2010, featuring radio, television, print advertising, and grassroots organizing to underscore the importance of having health insurance. Other organizations provided financial or in-kind support to the campaigns.

Chronic Illness Care

In the 1990s, as it became clear that chronic conditions such as asthma, diabetes, and depression were dominating health in the United States—accounting for more than three-quarters of the nation's health care expenditures—the Foundation developed a number of initiatives focused on improving the care of people with chronic illnesses. It approached the subject along three tracks.

The first consisted of programs to improve the way chronic care is delivered—particularly by managed care organizations, which in the 1990s were beginning to play a more important role in the health care landscape. Perhaps the most significant of these programs was "the chronic care model" pioneered by Edward Wagner, a physician with the Group Health Cooperative, a Seattle-based HMO. Wagner's model, which relies on teams of health care professionals working with patients to manage and monitor their chronic illnesses, has been widely adopted by HMOs throughout the country. The Foundation also tested, through a program called Cash & Counseling, the concept of giving homebound seniors the authority to control the way in which money was spent on their own personal care, even to the extent of paying family members rather than agencies.[36] Congress subsequently passed legislation permitting states to adopt this approach as an option within Medicaid.

The second chronic-care track supported initiatives to improve the *quality* of the care provided to people with chronic illnesses.[37] *The Dartmouth Atlas of Health Care*, which compares the quality and cost of care—especially chronic care—in different locales, has been particularly influential, as has research by Elizabeth McGlynn and her colleagues at RAND that found patients received recommended care only 55 percent of the time.[38] The Foundation funded two groups—the National Committee for Quality Assurance and the National Quality Forum—that set quality-of-care standards, particularly for chronic care, and certify health care organizations based on their compliance with the standards. Moreover, the Foundation tested ways that health care systems could adopt management practices from Toyota and other famously efficient companies, hospitals could reduce medical errors, and providers' pay could be linked with their performance.

The third track focused on improving care for individuals with such specific chronic illnesses as asthma, depression, and diabetes. The projects funded under these initiatives tended to focus on improving the systems of delivering care for these specific conditions.[39]

In addition to the three tracks, which tended to focus on improving systems of care for chronically ill people, the Foundation developed a large ($90 million) program, Faith in Action, that supported interfaith coalitions whose volunteers would deliver services to their homebound neighbors. At one point, more than a thousand interfaith coalitions were participating.

Looking Back at the Schroeder Years

When Schroeder arrived, he quickly refocused the Foundation on a limited number of objectives—tobacco and substance abuse, chronic care, and access to care. His longest lasting program legacy will probably be the Foundation's work to reduce smoking, followed closely by its work to bring palliative care into the medical mainstream. In both tobacco control and palliative care, the Foundation focused on policy change and used all of the tools available to philanthropy—research, advocacy, communications, evaluation, training, and convening—to reach its goals.

After the failure of the Clinton plan in 1994, national health reform dropped from the policy agenda. This, combined with the severe criticism of the Foundation for its suspected partisanship, led the Foundation to concentrate largely on state-level reforms and policy research during the rest of the decade. In terms of its chronic care priority, the Foundation did not enjoy great successes in the 1990s, but it kept a moral stake in the ground at a time when major change was unlikely. Many grantees funded by the Foundation in the 1990s—Dartmouth, the quality ratings agencies, and the Institute for Healthcare Improvement, for example—are now the leaders in the "quality movement" that has gained increasing importance in the 2000s.

Perhaps the most significant legacy of the Schroeder era was giving *health* an equal status with *health care*. During the Rogers presidency, the Foundation had focused almost exclusively on health care. In the Cluff era, there was some recognition of factors influencing health other than health care. With the research of J. Michael McGinnis and William Foege in the early 1990s showing that behavior and class had a more significant impact on health than medical care,[40] an increased emphasis on health made eminent good sense. But it was not an easy sell in a Foundation whose Board and staff were accustomed to viewing their role as improving health care.

Finally, Schroeder made a conscious effort to increase the Board's diversity and make it a truly national one. When he became the president in 1990, the Board was comprised of white males, nearly all of whom lived in New Jersey. When Schroeder left, the Board had members from around the country, and included an African American and a Latina. Four of the seventeen trustees were women.

—ᵕᵕ— The Risa Lavizzo-Mourey Era: 2003–Present

When Schroeder retired at the end of 2002, the Board, now chaired by former J&J vice chairman Robert Campbell (Tom Kean became the chairman in 2005), promoted Risa Lavizzo-Mourey from senior vice president for health care to president and chief executive officer.

A geriatrician by training and a health policy expert by experience, Lavizzo-Mourey, who had come to the Foundation from the University of Pennsylvania, retained the overall organizational structure of the Foundation, naming James Marks as the vice president for health and John Lumpkin to succeed her as the vice president for health care. She organized the Foundation's work around teams (currently, there are seven teams: human capital, vulnerable populations, coverage, quality/equality, public health, childhood obesity, and pioneer) that were charged with carrying out the strategic priorities established in a new Impact Framework. Lavizzo-Mourey made a public commitment of $500 million to reduce childhood obesity by 2015, and she has placed considerable emphasis on improving nursing care, expanding health insurance coverage, and improving the quality and equality of care. She has also developed the Foundation's brand, and with it has increased the Foundation's capacity to bring about social change and influence health policy.

Because Lavizzo-Mourey is still serving as president and CEO, it is premature to attempt to assess her legacy. An interview with her, as she looks back on her first decade as the Foundation's president, follows as the next chapter.

Notes

1. This and other quotes from Rogers were taken from his 1994 interview for the Foundation's oral history.

2. This and other quotes from Blendon were taken from his 1991 interview for the Foundation's oral history.

3. Rogers, D.E. Thoughts Regarding The Robert Wood Johnson Foundation's Public Affairs-Public Information Program," Report of the President and Staff to the Board of Trustees, May 24, 1973, p. 116.

4. Blendon, R. J., Aiken, L. H., and Rogers, D. E. "Improving Health and Medical Care in the United States: A Foundation's Early Experience." *The Journal of Ambulatory Care Management*, November 1983, 1–11.

5. Goodwin, P. Personal communication, 2011.

6. This and other quotes from Aiken were taken from her 1993 interview for the Foundation's oral history.

7. See Alper, J. "The Nurse Home Visitation Program." *To Improve Health and Health Care: The Robert Wood Johnson Foundation Anthology*, Vol. V. San Francisco: Jossey-Bass, 2002.

8. See Holloway, M. "The Regionalized Perinatal Care Program." *To Improve Health and Health Care: The Robert Wood Johnson Foundation Anthology*, Vol. IV. San Francisco: Jossey-Bass, 2001.

9. See Lear, J. G., Isaacs, S. L., and Knickman, J. R. *School Health Services and Programs*. San Francisco: Jossey-Bass, 2006.

10. This and other quotes from Cluff were taken from his 1991 interview for the Foundation's oral history.

11. This and other quotes from Cohen were taken from his 1993 interview for the Foundation's oral history.

12. The ten priority areas were: (1) infants, children, and adolescents, (2) chronic illness and disability, (3) AIDS, (4) destructive behavior, including substance abuse and violence, (5) mental illness, (6) organization and financing of health services, (7) quality of care, (8) ethical issues, including unequal access and the rising field of genetics, (9) health manpower, and (10) the impact of medical advances.

13. As quoted in Gardner, J. C. "The Robert Wood Johnson Foundation: 1974–2002." *To Improve Health and Health Care: The Robert Wood Johnson Foundation Anthology*, Vol. X. San Francisco: Jossey-Bass, 2006.

14. The Dementia Care and Respite Services program in 1986, which was replicated in 1992 with the Partners in Caregiving program.

15. Gardner, J. C. "The Robert Wood Johnson Foundation: 1974–2002." *To Improve Health and Health Care: The Robert Wood Johnson Foundation Anthology*, Vol. X. San Francisco: Jossey-Bass, 2006.

16. This and other quotes from Schroeder were taken from his 1995 and 2007 interviews for the Foundation's oral history.

17. SmokeLess States grantees were strictly forbidden from using the Foundation's funds for lobbying.

18. The Center for Public Program Evaluation. "The Tobacco Campaigns of the Robert Wood Johnson Foundation and Its Collaborators, 1991–2010." *RWJF Retrospectives Series*, http://www.rwjf.org/files/research/72051.tobaccocampaigns.050311.pdf, 2011.

19. Fighting Back, a program begun under the Cluff administration and expanded in the 1990s. See Wielawski, I. M. "The Fighting Back Program." *To Improve Health and Health Care: The Robert Wood Johnson Foundation Anthology*, Vol. VII. San Francisco: Jossey-Bass, 2004.

20. Free to Grow, on which the Foundation collaborated with the Doris Duke Charitable Foundation. See Wielawski, I. M. "Free to Grow." *To Improve Health and Health Care: The Robert Wood Johnson Foundation Anthology*, Vol. IX. San Francisco: Jossey-Bass, 2006.

21. See Solovitch, S. "Reclaiming Futures." *To Improve Health and Health Care: The Robert Wood Johnson Foundation Anthology*, Vol. XIII. San Francisco: Jossey-Bass, 2010.

22. See Parker, S. G. "Reducing Youth Drinking: The 'A Matter of Degree' and 'Reducing Underage Drinking through Coalitions' Programs." *To Improve Health and Health Care: The Robert Wood Johnson Foundation Anthology*, Vol. VIII. San Francisco: Jossey-Bass, 2005.

23. Ibid.

24. Paths to Recovery—jointly funded with the federal Center for Substance Abuse Treatment—focused, with some success, on reducing waiting times and no-shows and increasing admissions and continuation rates in substance-abuse treatment programs. Resources for Recovery helped states expand their substance-abuse treatment systems. In 2006 the Foundation funded a third program, Advancing Recovery, which sought to implement evidence-based practices in substance-abuse treatment through state-provider partnerships in twelve states.

25. Bornemeier, J. "The Robert Wood Johnson Foundation's Efforts to Combat Drug Addiction." *To Improve Health and Health Care: The Robert Wood Johnson Foundation Anthology*, Vol. XIII. San Francisco: Jossey-Bass, 2010.

26. Palliative care can be distinguished from end-of-life care in that it offers care to all seriously ill patients, whether or not they are dying.

27. Patrizi, P., Thompson, E., and Spector, A. "Improving Care at the End of Life: How the Robert Wood Johnson Foundation and Its Grantees Built the Field." *RWJF Retrospective Series*, www.rwjf.org/pr/product.jsp?id=71944, 2011.

28. The three programs were the Generalist Physician Initiative, under which thirteen medical schools tried to increase the number of generalists by revising curriculum, admissions, and teaching; the Generalist Physician Faculty Scholars Program, which awarded three-year grants to junior faculty members in primary care fields; and the Generalist Provider Research Initiative, which fostered research in primary care.

29. See Wielawski, I. M. "Practice Sights: State Primary Care Development Strategies." *To Improve Health and Health Care: The Robert Wood Johnson Foundation Anthology*, Vol. VI. San Francisco: Jossey-Bass, 2003.

30. See Wielawski, I. M. "Reach Out: Physicians' Initiative to Expand Care to Underserved Americans." *To Improve Health and Health Care 1997: The Robert Wood Johnson Foundation Anthology*. San Francisco: Jossey-Bass, 1997.

31. The Partnerships for Training program. See Green, L. "Improving Health Care in Rural America." *To Improve Health and Health Care: The Robert Wood Johnson Foundation Anthology*, Vol. XII. San Francisco: Jossey-Bass, 2009.

32. See Diehl, D. "The Southern Access Rural Program." *To Improve Health and Health Care: The Robert Wood Johnson Foundation Anthology*, Vol. X. San Francisco: Jossey-Bass, 2007.

33. This quote from Wentz was taken from his 1995 interview for the Foundation's oral history.

34. See Morone, J. A. "The Robert Wood Johnson Foundation and the Politics of Health Care Reform: Communications, Advocacy, and Policy Development." *To Improve Health and Health Care: The Robert Wood Johnson Foundation Anthology*, Vol. XII. San Francisco: Jossey-Bass, 2009.

35. See Rosenblatt, R. "The Robert Wood Johnson Foundation's Efforts to Cover the Uninsured." *To Improve Health and Health Care: The Robert Wood Johnson Foundation Anthology*, Vol. IX. San Francisco: Jossey-Bass, 2006. See also Nakashian, M. "Increasing Health Insurance Coverage at the Local Level: The Communities in Charge Program." *To Improve Health and Health Care: The Robert Wood Johnson Foundation Anthology*, Vol. X. San Francisco: Jossey-Bass, 2007.

36. The Cash and Counseling program. Benjamin, A. E., and Snyder, R. E. "Consumer Choice in Long-Term Care." *To Improve Health and Health Care: The Robert Wood Johnson Foundation Anthology*, Vol. V. San Francisco: Jossey-Bass, 2002.

37. See Newbergh, C. "Improving Quality of Care." *To Improve Health and Health Care: The Robert Wood Johnson Foundation Anthology*, Vol. XII. San Francisco: Jossey-Bass, 2009.

38. McGlynn, E. A., and colleagues. "The Quality of Health Care Delivered in the United States." *Journal of the American Medical Association*, 2003, *348*, 2635–2645.

39. See, for example, Levy, A. D. "The Robert Wood Johnson Foundation's Efforts to Address Pediatric Asthma." *To Improve Health and Health Care: The Robert Wood Johnson Foundation Anthology*, Vol. XII. San Francisco: Jossey-Bass, 2009.

40. McGinnis, J. M., and Foege, W. H. "Actual Causes of Death in the United States." *Journal of the American Medical Association*, 1993, *270*, 2207–2012.

CHAPTER 2

A Conversation with Risa Lavizzo-Mourey

Stephen L. Isaacs

—⁓— Background and Values

SI: You have written and spoken about the importance of social justice and the need for equity in health and health care. I imagine that these reflect values you developed when you were growing up. Would you talk a bit about your early years and upbringing?

RLM: I was born in Nashville, Tennessee, at the hospital affiliated with Meharry Medical College. My parents were in training there, my father in surgery and my mother in pediatrics. When I was two years old, they moved from Nashville to Seattle, partly because my father had a chance to be a surgical resident in the public health hospital and partly because they felt that life in the Northwest, without Jim Crow, would be a lot better than what they had experienced in the South. Plus my father loved the mountains and the water.

In a lot of ways, Seattle was a very progressive place. But there were still vestiges of the times—racism, and a real lack of social supports for people who were poor. My parents had a practice—as side-by-side solo practitioners, really—in the Central District, where most of the African Americans lived. It was a typical transition neighborhood; most new groups of people to Seattle lived there at one time or another. I spent a lot of time in my parents' office, one because I liked it and also because both of my parents were physicians with no child-care supports in Seattle so at times there was no other option. I recall the excitement when they would be called to the emergency room at night and my brother and I would go along and hang out at the nurses' station or in the waiting room while they saw their patients, and then we'd all go home.

As a result, I got a chance at a very early age to see how what we now call "social determinants"—issues of education and the economy and job security—affected health and people's willingness to seek health care.

SI: Beyond the influence of your parents, what else helped shape your values?

RLM: One of them was being part of the civil rights movement. As distant as it was from the South, we still had our version in Seattle. My mother was from Atlanta and she grew up in Ebenezer Baptist Church. Martin Luther King, Sr. married my parents and buried my grandparents. When Martin Luther King, Jr. came to Seattle to speak, he came to our house, and I got a chance to meet him—to spend time with this iconic figure and to absorb his values. The importance of being engaged in the movement, of fighting for civil rights and social justice, were themes in our household.

Another was seeing the importance of people having access to health care. I can remember a conversation with my mother in about 1968, when there was a recession in Seattle, and Boeing, one of the two major employers at the time, was laying people off. I overheard my parents talking about the patients who weren't coming in to get needed services because they had lost their insurance, and I remember asking naively what having a job or health insurance had to do with a person's decision to seek health care. And my mother breaking it down—how much people can afford to spend on things like health care and how much they had to reserve for other things. And how when people don't have health insurance, they are forced to make real choices between rent and medicine. I grew up hearing that and being influenced by it.

About that same time there was a mother of four named Odessa Brown, who had leukemia and was not able to get health care because she wasn't insured. When she died, the community rallied to build a community health center and named it after Odessa Brown. It's a clinic for kids based on the community-oriented primary care model, and my mother was its first medical director.

Thus, the broader issues of health and health care, social justice, and the importance of public health were part of my upbringing.

SI: When did you decide to become a physician, and a public health physician at that?

RLM: I always knew I was going to be a doctor, from the time I was three years old. I talked about it all the time, but became serious about it in middle school.

My father died the summer before I was to start at Yale, so I stayed in Seattle for my first year and attended the University of Washington. Since I was registering late, I had to scurry to find courses. As luck would have it, I wandered into the introductory course in public health. I hadn't thought about how influential that was on my thinking until recently when I was thumbing through the textbook, which I still have at home, and realized that the lectures in that course gave me a public health perspective—even before I had gotten a medical perspective.

A lot of my values came from my experiences as a Robert Wood Johnson Clinical Scholar, where after a long period of being focused on the traditional parts of medicine, I was reconnected with people who were thinking about health services research and broader issues of health and health care.

SI: How did you get to business school after receiving your medical degree?

RLM: My husband, Bob, and I had moved to Boston because I wanted to go to medical school at Harvard and then train at Brigham and Women's Hospital. When we finished our seven-year stint in Boston, it was my husband's turn to choose which city we lived in. (We had agreed that we were going to alternate choices of cities so that neither of us got a career advantage permanently.) He got a faculty job in Philadelphia so we moved to Philly. I had planned to get an MPH after my residency. It turned out, however, that Philadelphia did not have a school of public health. But there was a business school, Wharton, with an emphasis on health care administration and policy. Since I wanted to get a perspective on populations and analyzing the world in ways broader than the individual patient, I went to business school in health care administration. I began to see how my career could be broader than having a research career that focused upon an enzyme.

SI: Though you developed a broad interest in health policy, you specialized in geriatrics. What was behind that decision?

RLM: My main interest was in health policy, and I believed that Medicare was always going to drive health policy. Additionally, between finishing my residency at the University of Pennsylvania and starting the Clinical Scholars program, I had worked as a primary care physician at Temple in Philadelphia. I loved it but found it limiting in the sense that I had spent a lot of years learning how to take care of very sick and very complex patients, and most of the people I treated were young, relatively healthy women. The few geriatric patients that I had were both intellectually stimulating and very satisfying to treat. Following the academic medicine model, where your specialty should align with your research interest, I decided that aligning my interest in health policy with a research and clinical specialty in geriatrics made all the sense in the world for me.

SI: How did that alignment work out in practice?

RLM: I spent my time as a Robert Wood Johnson Clinical Scholar trying to bring the three worlds together: clinical medicine, academic medicine, and health policy—all with a focus on geriatrics. Since medical school, I had aspired for a career in academic medicine, so I stayed on at the University of Pennsylvania as an assistant professor. At the same time, I began to develop a relationship with the health policy community in Washington.

But bringing it all together—the things I had learned in business school such as setting goals and using measurement to drive the advancement of those goals and the values I had learned in medical school about caring for patients and understanding their needs—was a challenge. In fact, a colleague of mine, Allan Hillman, and I taught a course at Wharton for several years trying to bring these two cultures together. Trying to be a bridge between the multiple venues was a theme for me at the time—and still is.

SI: Then you went to Washington?

RLM: Late in the first Bush administration, the Agency for Health Care Policy and Research, now known as the Agency for Healthcare Research and Quality (AHRQ), was established. The Secretary of Health and Human Services, Louis Sullivan, and the administrator, Jarrett Clinton, approached me about becoming the deputy administrator. At the time, pundits were saying that health care reform was going to be a big issue in the next election; it was something that the Democrats wanted and it was also on President Bush's agenda. This agency was going to be involved in it, or so the word on the street said.

The position brought together all the things that I considered important. So against the advice of many of my academic colleagues, I went to Washington and commuted home to Philadelphia on the weekends for two years.

Within a year of my arriving at AHRQ, Bill Clinton was elected. When he started putting together work groups to lead his health care reform, he asked agencies for people who could go to the White House to work on it, and I was asked to go.

I spent a year and a half working at the White House, first with the quality work group and then as part of the communications team. Penn's policy dictated that after two years, I had to either re-up for another two years or return to the faculty full time. At that point, I had been commuting for two years and the time away from home and our young kids was tough; so I returned to Penn and academia. I used the platform of academia to work on the same issues, just with a much different perspective.

SI: How did you get to the Robert Wood Johnson Foundation?

RLM: I was moving along a wonderful trajectory at Penn and was starting to think about the next stage of my career. I had considered a number of leadership positions within academic medicine. After turning several down, it became clear to me that that wasn't what I wanted.

Out of the blue Steve Schroeder called me and said that the position of senior vice president for health care was open—would I be interested? Initially I said no, but fortunately Steve called me back a couple of days later and asked, "Are you sure you're comfortable with your decision?" "I've been rethinking it since you called me," I told him. "Why don't you come and talk to me?" he said.

That's how I got to the Foundation. Boy, am I glad that Steve called me back!

SI: As you look back, who would you say are the people who most influenced you?

RLM: I would put my mother first. She taught me the broader sense of how social determinants came into play and motivated me to be a doctor. Sam Martin and John Eisenberg at the University of Pennsylvania were important influences in how I thought about things like measurement in research and improving quality of care.

With exposure to leadership from a broader perspective, it was less the people I came into contact with and more the people whose leadership style I admired. For example, Nelson Mandela has talked about "leading from behind."* This approach suits my temperament, and I think that it has served the Foundation extremely well. It is also a style suitable for an organization that, as Steve Schroeder used to say, "doesn't deliver any health care services, doesn't make any products, doesn't regulate, and doesn't pay for it." So our role has to be very much an indirect one.

—ᗯᗯ— Goals and Strategies as the President and CEO of the Robert Wood Johnson Foundation

SI: When you became president in 2003, what did you hope to accomplish?

RLM: You'll recall that in 1999, the Foundation had divided into two program groups: the health care group, which focused on the delivery of medical care, and the health group which concentrated on the nonmedical factors, such as smoking and diet, that influence people's health. When I became president, the Foundation was still dealing with that reorganization. The people on the health side were concerned that they were never going to catch up to the health care side in terms of funding, and the people on the health care side questioned whether we needed to have this separation at all. I felt that we needed to develop a balanced yet integrated approach to health and health care. That was the stimulus for the Impact Framework.

Also, as a foundation, we were struggling with how we did our work and who we were. We still referred to ourselves as "grantmakers." We spoke about the importance of strategy, and about the importance of communications. But we hadn't put it together in a comprehensive way. By observing how the staff worked, I was able to develop "the five Cs" as a way of describing how we accomplished our objectives and created impact.

---

* *Editors' note*: The complete quote from Mandela is, "It is better to lead from behind and to put others in front, especially when you celebrate victory when nice things occur. You take the front line when there is danger. Then people will appreciate your leadership."

Third, I felt that we had been defined by major contributions in tobacco control and end-of-life care, and that we needed to have other areas that could similarly define us. So I began reading and talking to people about the big problems facing health and health care that others were not taking on in a major way.

SI: After you assumed office, the words "social change" were used frequently in describing the work of the Robert Wood Johnson Foundation. What do you mean by social change and why is it important?

RLM: The concept of social change goes back to our mission—"to improve health and health care for all Americans." The most important word to me is "improve." That's an action verb, and for us to improve health and health care, we have to look at social structures and the norms that our country abides by—and to change them. I look at social change as a transformative change that results in the lives of people being measurably better. I put the kinds of things that need to happen to improve health and health care on a par with other major social advances in this country, like civil rights and education reform.

SI: You mentioned earlier "the five Cs" as tools the Foundation uses to bring about social change. Could you describe the five Cs and why they are important for the Foundation?

RLM: In 2001, when I came to the Foundation, we were transitioning from thinking about ourselves primarily as grant-makers to thinking of ourselves as agents of social change. But although there was a lot of discussion about creating social change, we still talked mainly about our grantmaking and our grantees and getting money into the field. We didn't describe the other activities that we engaged in. For me, the five Cs were a way of summarizing what I heard the staff say they were doing here, about how we can use all of the tools available to philanthropy to create social change.*

---

* The five Cs are discussed in detail in chapter 4 of this volume.

It was clear that we spent a fair amount of time and resources on *communicating* results and doing it in a strategic way to get the information in the hands of the people who could make decisions. As part of everything we did we were always *convening*. We saw ourselves as a neutral convener. We were often the bridge *connecting* ideas and people. We also played a role in *coordinating* a lot of the different work, something we talked about frequently. And since I wanted to make it alliterative, I struggled with how to characterize evaluation and our commitment to measuring, and I came up with *counting*. Those five are all parts of the work that characterizes the Robert Wood Johnson Foundation. But because we were spending so much of our time talking about the cash (which could count as a sixth C), we weren't conscious of them.

SI: You also developed the Foundation's "Promise" shortly after you became president and CEO. Where did it come from and what is its significance?

RLM: The Promise was our way of talking about what we saw our brand to be—what distinguished us from others.* But the resistance from a lot of the staff led us to avoid the word "brand," which was seen as something that industry does. I remember some staff members saying, "We're not soap; we don't need a brand." So we developed another way to describe the concept of a brand, to tell our audience what differentiated us from others and what it is that we promise to do. We then went about a process to understand how others saw us and how we saw ourselves. Through that process, we came to understand that the field had a much better sense of what our promise was than we had internally. It was folks outside who said, "You take on the big, important things." "You have a rigorous approach to producing evidence that can be used for policy change." "You want to make a difference." We said, "That's what we try to do. We just never talk about it like that."

And that's how we came up with the Promise.

---

* The Promise is included as Appendix A.

SI: There is another, shorter document, the Foundation's "Guiding Principles." Why and how was this developed?

RLM: Early in his presidency, Steve Schroeder had developed a document that was called the Foundation's "Core Values"—patterned after the credo of Johnson & Johnson—that described our responsibilities to various constituencies. He developed it at the prompting of Jim Burke, a Board member and former CEO of J&J. As part of the interview process and of my study of the Foundation and J&J, I learned that when Burke became the chairman of J&J, he asked everybody to reexamine the company's credo. After a great deal of analysis and discussion, the J&J leadership recommitted to it. It's been written that the values expressed in the credo made it easy for J&J to do the right thing when the poisoning of Tylenol came along.

When I stepped into Steve's shoes, we were in a period of redefining ourselves. We had the Core Values document, but it was not as accessible as it should have been. So we engaged in a similar kind of exercise as J&J had. We had small groups examine the language, and then we had an active discussion throughout the Foundation. The result was our Guiding Principles, a document that represented what we aspired to do and how we aspired to conduct ourselves.* We put it on the wall and on everyone's desks, and we use it as our touchstone.

SI: At about the same time, you were developing an Impact Framework. How did this come about and what did you see as its purpose?

RLM: The Impact Framework is the way we conceptualize our programmatic work; it articulates our priorities. The concept of multiple portfolios, each with a set of characteristics that it tries to stay true to and which contribute to the overall mission, came out of our understanding of mutual funds. Just as mutual

---

* The Guiding Principles are included as Appendix B.

funds have different portfolios of funds for low-, medium-, and high-risk investments, the Foundation could also diversify *its* portfolios, though along program lines. The idea was that once you have these defined, you could dial them up or dial them down, depending on your assets, the external environment, and the probability of success.

—∿— The Foundation's Portfolios and Priorities

Childhood Obesity

SI: Let's turn to the Foundation's different portfolios and the different priorities. Perhaps we should start with childhood obesity—the one that is most public and most identified with your legacy.

RLM: When I became the Foundation's president, I was looking for an issue where the Foundation could have a significant impact on improving the nation's health, much as we have had in tobacco. Based on my research, two rose to the top—quality of care and childhood obesity. Another possibility was health insurance coverage, but at the time, an expansion of coverage seemed almost impossible. And we were still reeling from the defeat of health reform during the Clinton years.

Around the time I first joined the Foundation, the Surgeon General's report on obesity came out.[1] It said that childhood obesity was a largely underappreciated problem, one that had been accelerating for nearly a decade and a half and that no one was taking on directly. As I was preparing my first president's message, I remembered that report and thinking, "Tackling obesity would be perfect as an issue for the Robert Wood Johnson Foundation. It's a big challenge. It's hard. It's messy. And success would really improve the nation's health."

We had a series of meetings with the staff and with the Board about what it would mean to take on childhood obesity.

A lot of people were daunted by it. They questioned whether it wasn't mostly about personal responsibility for adults and whether beleaguered schools would be able to change and, say, add more physical activity and serve healthy food. In the end we agreed that we should explore what could be done about *childhood* obesity, which was rising to alarming levels. This is similar to the approach we'd adopted in tobacco: focus on children. And it built on things we were already doing, such as promoting physical activity and improving the built environment.

Next we discussed whether we should take a clinical approach or a prevention approach to the problem. Jim Marks, the senior vice president for health, insisted that we take a preventive approach. Then the childhood obesity team honed the strategy. We agreed to concentrate on an age group—schoolchildren— where we had a significant number of policy levers; to concentrate on the energy-in and energy-burned equation; and to attempt to influence that from a policy perspective. Our trustees reminded us of our obligation to focus our efforts on the most vulnerable populations.

SI: You declared that not only was the Foundation's goal to halt childhood obesity, it was to reverse it. And you committed a large sum, $500 million, to the effort. What prompted you to do this?

RLM: I said we needed to have a goal, by a specific date. The childhood obesity team wrestled with this and concluded that the first thing we could do is to halt the rise. But Jim Marks said, "No, that's not good enough. We've got to reverse it." I then stuck our collective neck out by making it public. My reasoning went like this: I knew roughly how much money we were likely to spend on various large childhood obesity efforts. So rather than retrospectively saying, "We spent $500 million to combat childhood obesity," why not say in advance, "We are going to spend $500 million on childhood obesity." If the Foundation said that, others would sit up and think, "This is clearly a big problem, one deserving of the nation's attention."

So we announced a commitment of $500 million to reverse childhood obesity.

SI: How do you think things have been going and what big challenges are left?

RLM: I feel very good about how much progress the nation has made. With a problem like this, the first thing you have to do is to raise awareness and get a common agreement on the nature of the problem and an approach to solutions. It would be hard to find very many circles in which people don't see this as important. No matter whom you talk to—people in the military, business leaders, school administrators, cab drivers—everyone understands the importance of the issue. There's also a great appreciation about how the solutions require work across sectors. People acknowledge the important role of parents, but they also understand that business, urban planning, transportation, schools, and communities have to be involved. Today, there is an appreciation that just wasn't there in 2001 or even in 2003.

There are now pockets of real hope, in the sense of communities seeing a downturn in, or even reversals of, childhood obesity rates. Childhood obesity in Arkansas has gone down. California has documented a reversal of childhood obesity in some places. New York City; Philadelphia; El Paso, Texas; West Virginia; and Mississippi have seen successes as well. The Healthy Schools program, which takes a comprehensive approach, is demonstrating a decrease in body mass index (BMI).

A lot still needs to be done. First, we've got to get beyond isolated pockets of hope. Second, we have to address clinical needs in addition to preventive needs. Otherwise, we'll lose a whole cohort of kids who are already overweight or obese. Then the business case needs to be continually made to the food manufacturers. These, along with structural changes in our environment and incentives in how we spend our days, will sustain the reductions in childhood obesity we're beginning to see.

Even though there remains a lot to do, the fact that change is taking place in some areas—in a relatively short period of time—is enormously positive. In comparison to the length of time it took the tobacco-control community to start showing change, this is a much more accelerated time frame. I feel very good about that.

Coverage and Access to Care

SI: Expanding health insurance coverage and increasing access to care have been Foundation priorities since day one. The Foundation was active in the efforts to enact health care reform in the early 1990s, and received some criticism for its activism. What did the Foundation learn from that period and what did it do differently in 2009–2010?

RLM: Recognizing that a major policy change such as health care reform is a long-term proposition and that there is always going to be opposition, we maintained a strictly nonpartisan approach. We knew we were going to be in it for the long haul and that we would have to work across the aisle. So we developed principles of coverage but did not endorse any one approach to achieving them. We supported research that spoke to both sides. The consciously nonpartisan approach that we took, the principles for coverage that we developed, and the relationships formed with people across sectors—such as business and labor, insurance companies, and consumer advocacy groups (what we called the "strange bedfellows")—came out of our having been perceived as being aligned with groups that had a particular agenda in the 1990s.

At the same time, we know that expanded health insurance coverage is something that Democrats advocate more than Republicans. Cost reduction and quality improvement, on the other hand, are issues that often get bipartisan support. Our work on quality, particularly outside the Beltway, has been enormously helpful to our reputation as an organization looking to find solutions. And our support of activities both on the ground and at the federal level has added to our credibility.

SI: Now that the Affordable Care Act has passed, how is the Foundation positioning itself?

RLM: We've set a goal of having 95 percent of the people enrolled in insurance by 2020. The other big issue for us is cost. As a country, we are going to have to come to grips with the need to provide higher value care: better outcomes for the amount of money we're spending. We are building into our work an increasing emphasis on cost and value.

Similarly, we've started looking within our human capital portfolio at the policy questions vis-à-vis the workforce that must be addressed. This isn't saying that we're going to develop more fellowship or scholarship programs. Rather, we want to be engaged in helping develop policy solutions that will allow us to address the need for additional health care workers, especially primary care professionals, required to care for so many newly insured Americans.

Quality/Equality

SI: Why did you create a team that links quality and equality?

RLM: We have a long history of attempting to eliminate or decrease disparities, going back to the days of our first president, David Rogers. We funded programs to train minority faculty members and to help minority students, and we saw increasing access as a way of reducing disparities. I was on an Institute of Medicine committee that looked specifically at how to reduce disparities in the health care system. One of the conclusions of that committee was that quality improvement might be a way to reduce disparities. As president of the Foundation, I wanted to act on this IOM report. As we were going through the process of honing in on fewer strategic objectives, the idea that we could create a bridge between the two communities by linking quality improvement and disparities was a natural for us.

SI: What have been the priorities of the quality/equality team and how do you feel about the progress in achieving them?

RLM: Quality is another of those areas that has been on the Foundation's radar screen for a long time—and where success has proven elusive. In the 1990s, we gave a great deal of attention to developing the tools to measure quality and the organizations to set and uphold quality standards: The Joint Commission, the National Committee for Quality Assurance, and the National Quality Forum. I think that these, plus our support of *The Dartmouth Atlas* and the quality team at Dartmouth, have paid dividends. Now, we are mainly focused on improving quality on the ground through our Aligning Forces for Quality program, which is working with providers, payers, and consumers in sixteen locations. It's still too early to tell what impact the program will have, but the early reports are encouraging. And with the exception of the last eighteen months, health care costs have continued to rise, making it more important than ever to find ways of providing, and paying for, care based on its value.

Public Health

SI: How would you assess the Foundation's work to improve public health?

RLM: Public health was one of the teams that came about as the result of several different areas merging: our ongoing tobacco-control work and the incipient work shoring up the public health infrastructure. Bringing the two areas of work together was a struggle at first. We are now looking broadly at what we need to do to put prevention more firmly on the national agenda and to build an infrastructure to support that effort. The rewarding part of this is that people in the fields of public health and prevention have appreciated the fact that the Robert Wood Johnson Foundation has highlighted the importance of what they are doing and is getting more people to pay attention to their work. So I think that's been successful.

What's different about our priorities in public health compared with some of the other portfolios is their breadth. Therefore,

it's a little harder to define success. We've defined it as moderniz-
ing the public health system, but as we've heard in the midcourse
review of our public health programs, it's not clear to the field
exactly what success will look like.

Human Capital

SI: As you look back on the Foundation's work to develop
human capital, which dates back to 1972, what is your feeling
about its impact and where do you see it going?

RLM: I think that it is one of our most successful areas, if not
the most successful one. When you look at how external groups
rate us, human capital always comes out at the top. When we talk
to former fellows, they often tell us that the fellowship transformed
their career. Another measure that we look at is the percentage of
the top positions in American medicine filled by former Robert
Wood Johnson Foundation fellows. The percentage is very high,
something like 37 percent.

The strength of the human capital team is the three thousand
fellows and other alumni. I would like our network of former
fellows to become as valuable to us as alumni are to universities—a
pool of people who really are our reputational capital. Internally,
we are still trying to figure out the best ways to draw on that
enormous resource, and I want us to focus on that over the next
few years.

I should also signal our work in nursing, which is a priority of
the human capital team, as it has been for the Foundation since
its earliest days and was for our founder, Robert Wood Johnson.
Over the years, we've sought to strengthen the profession from a
wide range of angles—training nursing leaders, strengthening care
at the hospital bedside, and supporting research, among others.
Most recently, we funded the report of the Institute of Medicine
on *The Future of Nursing*. The report emphasizes the critical role
that nurses play in improving the quality of patient care and
provides a comprehensive platform for the full participation of

nurses. We recognize that this will take time, and we are in it for the long haul.

Vulnerable Populations

SI: Turning to vulnerable populations, how would you describe the work of the vulnerable populations team and how has it evolved?

RLM: When I first came to the Foundation, we talked about areas that were strategic and other areas that were opened up by people who were good at prospecting—people such as Terry Keenan, who were able to find those really great programs, the nuggets that needed to be developed, and who would then foster them. But because this kind of programming wasn't seen as strategic, a lot of people at the Foundation did not consider it to be valuable.

At the same time, we were always talking about how to take projects to scale. What the vulnerable populations team has defined as its niche is the perfect blend of the two—finding the nuggets and providing the additional resources to take them to a bigger scale. Programs like Playworks[2] and Green House[3] are well on their way. There are going to be others that won't get that far but which, with our help, will grow and serve many more people. Thus, we are using our skills to identify innovative programs that address the social determinants of health, and we are nurturing those programs and taking them to scale, in the ultimate hope of finding other partners that will continue supporting them. I think the vulnerable populations portfolio has been a great success.

Pioneer

SI: Last, but not least, how do you view the work of the pioneer portfolio?

RLM: Pioneer is the newest of all of our concepts. It has defined what it means to invest in something that is truly innovative—something that brings an approach from a different industry to health or health care and has the potential to change dramatically how we do our work—ideas such as Project ECHO or the OpenNotes program or, a few years ago, Games for Health.

Where we've struggled is in connecting the ideas that emerge from the pioneer portfolio with some of the other things we're doing. For example, we have a strategy in childhood obesity, but there is a lot going on related to childhood obesity that doesn't fit within that strategy, some of which could be real game changers—like some of the Games for Health, for example. If you were to get some of those games in schools, it could revolutionize the way kids get physical activity.

Project ECHO is another.[4] I remember ten years ago, we were struggling with the problem that poor people were not getting specialty care. One of the things that struck me in the Project ECHO video is that Sanjeev Arora, who developed the idea, said that there are shortages of specialists everywhere in the world. And when I heard Dr. Arora lead with that, I thought, "Here's something that has been a problem for a long time, and he has a very innovative way of dealing with it." We didn't come at it by saying to the pioneer team, "Here's the problem we're trying to fix—lack of specialty services in underserved areas. What can you do to solve that?" It just happened that way. I'd like to see it happen more frequently.

I'd like to see the pioneer team identify areas that might become important priorities for the Foundation in the future. It would be a great story if ten years from now we are moving in a new direction because of a little tiny something that we explored in the pioneer portfolio.

Enterprise-Level Programming

SI: Let's talk about enterprise-level programming. What is the "enterprise level" and what is its purpose?

RLM: It gets back to some of the early concerns expressed after we divided the Foundation into health and health care groups: that we were never going to take on big areas that don't fall neatly into one or another team. That we were not going to be a single foundation any longer. The enterprise-level programs address those concerns.

A lot of the work we think is important doesn't fall neatly within one team or another. This kind of work, which cuts across teams, we have termed our enterprise-level work because it involves the enterprise—the Foundation—as a whole. There are many examples. Take, for example, reducing health care costs. It has implications for our work in quality, coverage, prevention, and vulnerable populations, and yet none of those teams can concentrate on it, so it becomes an enterprise effort. We envisioned enterprise as an opportunity for someone who has a really great idea that addresses the enterprise as a whole to write it up and present it to senior management. If it's approved, that person can oversee the program.

We've always had enterprise-level work, like *Health Affairs*, Grantmakers In Health, The Center for Effective Philanthropy, and the National Health Policy Forum—even the *Anthology*. We have simply identified it and given it a name.

Impact Capital

SI: Related to these points, there has been much talk in philanthropy about the use of "impact capital," that is, nontraditional ways of funding programs. How has the Foundation used this and what do you see as its future?

RLM: One of the things I've noticed is that some philanthropies working in other social areas employ their capital more adventurously than we in health and health care do. If you look at education or the environment, foundation leaders are talking about using mission-related investments and double- or triple-bottom-line investing. In health and health care, we have been relatively limited to grants. The Robert Wood Johnson Foundation has done some program-related investments, but not very many.[5] One of our challenges is to use these diverse financing mechanisms more effectively.

—w— Evaluation and Communications

SI: The Foundation has always given great importance to evaluation. Would you describe how you view its role currently and in the future?

RLM: I think evaluation has evolved in interesting ways, and the research and evaluation unit is in the process of defining a different role for itself as the Foundation has become more focused. We've done program-by-program evaluations, and we've examined clusters of programs as the *Anthology* does. We're now working with two innovations. First, we are doing midcourse reviews of some of our strategies. Based on what we find, we can make adjustments in the programs or the balance among programs. Second, we are looking at how we've done in a body of work that has largely closed—what we call "retrospectives." We've done retrospectives on chronic illness, tobacco, end-of-life care, and substance abuse. When we start to integrate what we've found from all of the retrospectives, there are going to be some very interesting lessons for the Foundation and for philanthropy in general.

Second, we are adopting new methods, such as network analysis, in ways that are still to be played out but that I find very encouraging. We are continuing to ask ourselves if we can develop methods that will allow us to quantify the value of our work in more efficient, more rigorous ways than we've done before. Those are new approaches to evaluation that could be interesting and exciting for the field.

SI: And communications?

RLM: I believe that we have defined the field of strategic communications within the nonprofit and philanthropic areas. Tobacco was the success story. Close behind is coverage; we did a lot in coverage that others didn't have the wherewithal to do.

Now, we're defining how we can be strategic with a much larger audience.

We have always felt that because our resources were limited, we couldn't afford to reach out to many people beyond the policymaking and stakeholder elites. But with the concept of Web 2.0 and social media, we are revisiting that. I'm not sure how it's going to play out, but I believe we now have the opportunity to reach many more people in a very strategic way than we had, say, fifteen years ago. For me, that is the great challenge for communications.

Assessing the Impact Framework and Team Programming

SI: In retrospect, how do you think the Impact Framework and team programming have worked?

RLM: I don't think we're going to be able to say how well it's worked until we've been through a complete cycle of a set of strategic objectives. But on the whole, I think it has worked pretty well. An issue for us has been that the teams managing the three nontargeted portfolios—human capital, vulnerable populations, and pioneer—have struggled with what their real purpose is. They wanted to be like the targeted portfolios.

The vulnerable populations team has gotten beyond that and has defined who it is and how it's going to operate. The team is clear about what it does, and this is gratifying. The pioneer portfolio has given us a window into a great many interesting things. I don't think we would be as far along on our Web 2.0 philanthropy thinking if it weren't for the pioneer team. Nor would we have gotten into some really innovative projects like Games for Health and the OpenNotes project. The pioneer portfolio is still young. Its history is yet to be written.

Human capital offers an example of our ability to dial up and dial down, depending on the circumstances. Between 2000 and 2003, we had a huge budget for our coverage portfolio, but when it looked like we weren't going to get anywhere with expanding coverage, we started reducing that budget and putting more into human capital programs. Now we're increasing coverage again and reducing human capital, which is painful. It's not easy to dial things up and down. That's a lesson we've learned.

Another lesson we've learned is that in the targeted portfolios, we've got to be really targeted. Four targeted priorities are probably about all you can handle.

—ᴡ— Management and Governance

SI: Related to these points, I would like to get your views on managing the Foundation. Would you talk about the pros and cons of the team approach and how it's evolved over time?

RLM: The concept evolved from being a group of people who did their individual programming while *calling themselves* a team to one where there really *is* a team. The change had to do with two things. The first was requiring teams to develop an objective with some measurements related to it. We had a couple of periods when we had to cut back on resources and when the objective and the team's willingness to stick with it really had to be tested. Second, we gave real authority to the team director. Giving team directors the authority to make funding decisions and having people report to them brought decision making a lot closer to where strategic discussions were taking place.

The pros, I think, are that we have more programs that are on-strategy and the teams are very productive. The cons are, first of all, the risk of the Foundation becoming fragmented by teams; that's part of the reason we began to concentrate on the enterprise as a whole. Second, it doesn't reward those really creative, gifted program officers who are kind of Lone Rangers and who you don't want to stifle. I'm not sure that the likes of Terry Keenan would have done well on a team.

SI: How are you avoiding, or minimizing, the downsides of a team approach?

RLM: The answer to the first danger, fragmentation, is our enterprise-level programming. We have deliberately kept enterprise-level funding small because we don't want it to be a big part of what we do. At the same time, we want to provide an opportunity for those people who've got that creative spirit and see things in a broad perspective.

With regard to the second, nurturing innovative thinkers, we try to foster creativity in two ways. The first is through our pioneer portfolio. Pioneer is really a team made up of individuals who are good at prospecting. The other way, as I mentioned, is through our enterprise-level activities.

SI: Turning to governance, what do you see as the appropriate role for Board and staff, and how has it evolved over the years?

RLM: When I became the Foundation's president, one trustee described the role of the trustees as that of being a super program officer. The trustees made it clear to me after a retreat that they wanted the Board to be more focused on strategy and policy and less on individual programs.

We've largely achieved that. Most of the time, the Board talks about our overall strategy, our program strategies, and our progress in meeting our objectives. We only occasionally highlight individual programs. I believe that this is the appropriate role for the Board.

At the staff level, we tend to cluster things a lot more, by team and by strategic area. The downside is that people want to do more things by team and don't want to bring ideas to the entire program staff. There is a tension between, on the one hand, wanting to share information so that we function as a single foundation and, on the other hand, keeping decision making close enough to the people who know the material best. That tension will always exist.

One of the things that is a challenge and that I didn't fully appreciate going into this—or even until fairly recently—is that we now have a Board with term limits, and we're almost to the point where we've replaced the Board completely. We are no longer going to have long-serving trustees who are on the Board for fifteen, sixteen, or seventeen years and have a great deal of institutional memory. It's not happening anymore. But it's important that the Board, even though limited by terms, feels a deep connection to the Foundation.

SI: How do you get that connection? And how do you get a Board with such political diversity to agree on controversial topics, such as health care reform?

RLM: First of all, you seek Board members with a commitment to the Foundation's mission and work. I've learned that it is very important to choose people who have a history with the Foundation. Have they been a fellow? Do they know us through J&J and a commitment to Robert Wood Johnson? Have we funded them in the past? Have they had a connection as one of our collaborators? Are they from an organization that knows our work and shares our values? It's hard to come into an organization like ours as a trustee if you don't have something that connects you in that way. And, of course, we look for Board members who value our nonpartisan approach that seeks to find common ground.

Also, I spend a lot of time talking with the trustees, one on one, over the phone or in person. I try to visit them at least once every couple of years, in their own communities. When something arises that has the potential to be divisive or set a new policy, we set up a working group where we lay out and adopt general principles. Then, when it comes to the specifics of a project, the Board and staff have something to refer to for guidance. A good example is coverage. While our trustees had different views about how to achieve expanded insurance coverage, they all agreed with our principles that provided us with a framework for looking at health care reform—principles stating, for example, that everybody ought to have coverage and that care should be accessible and affordable.

—⚬— The Role of Philanthropy

SI: As you look back over ten years, what have you learned about the potential for and limitations of philanthropy in bringing about social change?

RLM: Foundations have a serious limitation, of course: we cannot lobby. As a result, we can't be as aggressive on particular issues as we might want to be. We get outspent and outmaneuvered in those kinds of situations all the time. Throughout the health care reform debates, which were pretty intense, we had to be quiet. That is the way Congress designed it, but it is enormously frustrating, when you have a good sense of the literature and you know the issues, to have to sit on your hands.

It is interesting how, over the past forty years, philanthropy has become increasingly transparent. We've helped make it like that. For example, publicly announcing our program goals and targets for 2015 is going to be a first for us and I think for any foundation. Once we've announced these, we will have to share publicly our assessment of how well we've done against them. In the past, when we changed directions, we were not quite as open as we are going to have to be in the future. It has forced me to think about how to do it, in a way that will serve both us and the field well.

The great potential of foundations is that they can choose difficult problems, stick with them for a long time, bring people to the table who wouldn't ordinarily come to it, and eventually, get things done that other sectors won't or can't. That's a real upside.

—⟋⟍— Appendix A: The Robert Wood Johnson Foundation Promise

We believe that good health and health care are essential to the well-being and stability of our society, the vitality of our families and communities, and the productivity of our economy—indeed, they are fundamental measures of our success as a nation.

Helping all Americans lead healthier lives and get the care they need is the mission of our Philanthropy. Our strategy is to identify major health challenges, seek bold, transformative solutions, and sustain our commitments until success is achieved. Our guiding principles flow from a sense of responsibility to all our constituents. In particular:

- To the nation, we pledge to tackle the greatest challenges to good health and health care for as long as it takes to achieve lasting results.

- To the most vulnerable among us, we pledge to pursue solutions that are effective, affordable, and equitable.

- To our grantees and collaborators, we pledge to set clear goals, forge strong and creative partnerships, and measure our work by transparent, evidence-based criteria that meet the highest standards of performance and integrity.

Through our actions we pledge an unyielding commitment to the philanthropic vision of our founder, General Robert Wood Johnson, whose remarkable business career and passion for improved health and health care made this work possible.

This promise is made by the trustees and staff of the Robert Wood Johnson Foundation.

—⟋⟍— Appendix B: Guiding Principles

Our mission is to improve the health and health care of all Americans. Thus, our fundamental responsibility is to help improve the conditions, policies and practices that protect and promote health and to improve the care people receive. Our philanthropy represents a public trust:

- We are stewards of private resources that must be used in the public's interest and particularly to help the most vulnerable in our society.

As investors in and partners with other organizations, we depend for our success on our grantees and our colleagues in the fields of health and health care and related disciplines. We must promote new ideas by encouraging innovation:

- We must select grantees fairly.
- We must be responsive to our grantees and to the field.
- We must be objective, rigorous, and transparent in assessing grantees' progress and the results of their work.
- We must communicate clearly and openly to the field and to the public.

Improving health and health care for all Americans depends on the performance of our staff at all levels:

- We must meet the highest professional and ethical standards.
- We must share a passionate dedication to our mission.
- We must commit ourselves to lifelong learning and continual improvement.
- We must represent different perspectives and experiences.
- We must respect the views of others.

Notes

1. *The Surgeon General's Call to Action to Prevent and Decrease Obesity and Overweight*, 2001.
2. See Newbergh, C. "Playworks/Sports4Kids." *To Improve Health and Health Care: The Robert Wood Johnson Foundation Anthology*, Vol. XIV. San Francisco: Jossey-Bass, 2011.
3. See Wielawski, I. M. "The Green House Program." *To Improve Health and Health Care: The Robert Wood Johnson Foundation Anthology*, Vol. XIV. San Francisco: Jossey-Bass, 2011.
4. See Solovitch, S. "Project ECHO," chapter 9 of this volume.
5. See Goodwin, P. and Navarro, M. "Program-Related Investments." *To Improve Health and Health Care: The Robert Wood Johnson Foundation Anthology*, Vol. V. San Francisco: Jossey-Bass, 2002.

CHAPTER 3

Terrance Keenan: An Appreciation

Digby Diehl

Editors' Introduction

Terry Keenan was the most beloved and effective grantmaker in the Foundation's history. A kind and gentle man who never said a bad word about anybody, Keenan had the tenacity of a terrier. He is legendary for having braved dangerous ghettos in Chicago and Arctic snows in Alaska in search of extraordinary grantees and then fighting for them, sometimes against great opposition, at the Robert Wood Johnson Foundation. He never gave up on an idea or a person he believed in. Alan Cohen, a former vice president of research and evaluation at the Foundation, said that Terry was "the social conscience of the Foundation" and "really sees the people in the project."

In his more than thirty-year career, Keenan championed and supervised nearly a thousand grants, many awarded to small community-based organizations. He was an early and impassioned advocate of the nursing profession and was instrumental in the Foundation's early efforts to build the field of nurse practitioners.

Even after his formal retirement in 2003, Keenan continued to serve the Foundation as a special program consultant, coming to work nearly every day until his death in 2009. His legacy continues in his influence on the field and through the Terrance Keenan Institute for Emerging Leaders in Health Philanthropy established by Grantmakers In Health.

In Volume IX of the *Anthology*, Digby Diehl wrote an appreciation of Keenan, one that captured—to the extent that they can be captured in a short piece—his life and values. We reprint that appreciation here, both as a tribute to, and as a way of sharing the philosophy of, a person who represents the very best of philanthropy.

—ɯ— **I**f you visit Terry Keenan at his modest home in the small village of Newtown, Pennsylvania, you are struck by how much the man lives up to his legend. Throughout the world of philanthropy, and particularly in the realm of health care philanthropy, Keenan is respected as a pioneer of modern grantmaking and a model program officer. He is a man who helped change both the reality and perception of foundations by greatly influencing the development of contemporary grantmaking and foundation policy. As one of the original members of the Robert Wood Johnson Foundation staff in 1972, he played an important role in the institution for more than thirty years.

What is less known about Keenan is that he was the unlikely Indiana Jones of the Robert Wood Johnson Foundation. Keenan fearlessly ventured single-handed into urban jungles and traveled to remote rural outposts to bring health care to communities that were deeply in need. Like the movie character, he used his sharp intellect and academic training to analyze problems and find solutions. With no need of a whip or a gun, Keenan made his shy smile and friendly handshake the face of a giant foundation in small towns and struggling inner-city health projects throughout the country. He is revered as the man who took philanthropy out of the wood-paneled boardrooms and into the narrow alleys, the dirt roads, and the backwaters of America, where the most vulnerable populations needed help.

Keenan, who officially retired in December 2003, continues to be an influence at the Foundation as a special program consultant. At his home, he wears the same tan windbreaker for which he was well known at the Foundation, with the slight modification of a plaid flannel shirt instead of a white shirt and tie. Keenan is slight of build, perhaps five feet two inches tall. Wisps of white hair grace his otherwise bald head. He wears rimless glasses tinted yellow. Even behind the tinted lenses, his eyes flash with energy and enthusiasm as he speaks, and throughout the conversation he maintains the sort of eye contact and intensity that make you feel that his mission is to persuade you personally. He is no orator, but his manner expresses integrity and thoughtfulness. He repeats many of his noted precepts of grantmaking with an enthusiasm that is fresh and contagious.

If there is a single key to Keenan's extraordinary career in philanthropy, it is a booklet he wrote in 1992, *The Promise at Hand.*[1] This booklet is based on a series of lectures he gave at the Foundation in 1990–1991 as part of its twentieth-anniversary celebration. As Steven Schroeder, who was then the president and chief executive officer of the Foundation, wrote in his introduction, *The Promise at Hand* is "a distillation of the insights developed in [Keenan's] long and fruitful career."

What Makes a Foundation Great?

1. A great foundation is informed and animated by moral purpose.

2. A great foundation accepts responsibility and stewardship for pursuing these purposes.

3. A great foundation walks humbly with its grantees—it acknowledges that their success is the instrument of its own success.

4. A great foundation is deliberate. It is guided by judgment. It acts where there is a need to act. It takes necessary risks—and proceeds in the face of great odds.

5. A great foundation is a resource for both discovery and change. It invests not only in the identification of answers, but also in the pursuit of solutions.

6. A great foundation is accountable. It functions as a public trust—and places its learning and experience in the public domain.

7. A great foundation builds investment partnerships around its goals, creating coalitions of funders—public and private—to multiply its impact.

8. Conversely, a great foundation participates in funding coalitions being organized by other parties to lend its support to purposes requiring multiple funders.

9. Finally, a great foundation is self-renewing. It adheres to a constant process of self-reflection and self-assessment. It knows when it needs to change and to adopt measures to improve its performance.

—Terrance Keenan, *The Promise at Hand*

Because Keenan is, in Schroeder's words, "a living embodiment of the best aspects of the Robert Wood Johnson Foundation," his precepts for active philanthropy and foundation ethics in the booklet also reflect his personal standards.

—〰— Early Life

Keenan's diversified early career prepared him surprisingly well for grantmaking. He grew up in the bustling artistic community of New Hope, Pennsylvania, the son of Peter Keenan, a Modernist artist of the New Hope School, and a mother who ran the local tearoom. "My father had studied at the Slade School of Fine Art in London, and to support his serious painting—and his five children—he became a sports illustrator for the *Philadelphia Bulletin*," Keenan recalls. "He loved the surroundings of New Hope and the company of the other artists there. The American Impressionist painter John Fulton Folinsbee was one of our neighbors."

He began to follow in his father's artistic footsteps at age ten, when he was selected to exhibit his artwork at a local showing. World War II exposed him to the wider world; he spent the years 1944 to 1946 as a naval aviator, flying as a navigator throughout the South Pacific. When he returned to civilian life, he enrolled at Yale to study English literature. "Yale accepted almost three times as many students as usual in my class [of 1950] because of all the veterans," Keenan notes. "We were doubled up in rooms and the classes were crowded, but I loved the rich learning experiences." He graduated with Phi Beta Kappa honors and pursued each of his interests with such eclecticism that he qualified to teach English, Spanish, French, history, and art appreciation at the Thomas Jefferson prep school in St. Louis, Missouri, for the next five years. He even found time in his youth to become a Golden Gloves boxing contender. Laughing, Keenan insists modestly, "I wouldn't make too much of that. In my weight class, at 145 pounds, you just had to be fast and light on your feet and strong. You really didn't hurt anyone, and no one ever hurt me too badly."

When Keenan moved to New York, in 1955, he worked for the investment firm Merrill Lynch, Pierce, Fenner & Beane, where he was charged with writing the biography of the company's founder, Charles E. Merrill. A year later, exactly ten years after separating from the Navy, he began his long career in philanthropy as a writer for the Ford Foundation, directing the foundation's Office of Reports, under J. Quigg Newton. He joined the Ford Foundation the year it made a groundbreaking blanket distribution of $660 million to all colleges, universities, hospitals, and medical schools in the United States. As Paul Jellinek, a friend and former vice president at the Robert Wood Johnson Foundation, once joked, "For those of you who wonder where Terry got the idea of thinking about scale and thinking big, it started with $660 million from the Ford Foundation."[2] Among his many contributions at Ford, he was chief staff assistant to a trustees committee that wrote a visionary program for the expansion of the foundation in the 1960s.

—ᘉᘉ— Health Care Philanthropy

Health care philanthropy first beckoned to Keenan in May 1965, when he became senior executive associate and Board secretary of the Commonwealth Fund. As assistant to Quigg Newton, who had become the fund's president, he was involved with every phase of Commonwealth's activities. "Terry was Quigg's right-hand man, his scribe at the meetings and writer of everything for the foundation from the press releases to the annual reports," says Margaret Mahoney, a longtime friend and colleague of Keenan's. Mahoney is a former vice president of the Robert Wood Johnson Foundation, where she worked with Keenan, president emeritus of the Commonwealth Fund, and currently president of MEM Associates. "When we met, I had an executive associate position at the Carnegie Corporation similar to Terry's, and we became friends almost immediately," she recalls. "I was impressed that his grasp of the big health care issues was deepened by a genuine compassion for the recipients of health care. I think of him as a combination of the sharp-minded Jesuit and the caring parish priest."

What brought Mahoney from Carnegie and Keenan from Commonwealth together was a conference at the Massachusetts Institute of Technology in the late 1960s on the problems of medical care for the indigent. "The Carnegie Corporation gave the president of MIT $15 thousand to convene a conference on health care for the poor," Mahoney recalls. "Frankly, MIT did not have much interest in medical care or medicine at the time. All of the university medical centers were ignoring this huge problem, and our cities were burning. The report from that meeting more or less confirmed what we already knew. But it brought Carnegie and Commonwealth together to work on the problem. That's how I met Terry."

Frank Karel, former Robert Wood Johnson Foundation vice president for communications, recalls meeting Keenan for the first time in 1965, when he was head of public relations for Johns Hopkins Medical Institutions. "One day, the dean of the medical school, Tommy Turner, called to say that he had to meet with Quigg Newton from the Commonwealth Fund about a grant proposal, and Quigg was bringing some new staff member," Karel says. "The dean wanted me to get this new guy out of the room so that he could be alone with Quigg. That day, I took Terry on the $50 tour of Johns Hopkins, which was a huge sprawling place that covered about five city blocks. We went from the top of every building down into the tunnels below, and Terry loved it. He never stopped asking questions. Terry and I became friends, and the dean got his grant." Two years later, Karel joined Keenan at the Commonwealth Fund as a program officer, and he recalls that they were both struck by how completely independent, arrogant, and disorganized foundations were at that time. "The foundation world was really in disarray," Karel recalls. "They weren't organized; they didn't work together. Terry and I talked about the need for greater responsibility, accountability. This later led Terry to support the evaluation ethic that was championed at the Robert Wood Johnson Foundation from its earliest days. Of course, just a few years after we discussed the problem, Congress took an even dimmer view of foundations in the Tax Reform Act of 1969."

In addition to his concern for the structure and administration of foundations, Keenan began to focus on programmatic areas that would be lifelong pursuits. At the Commonwealth Fund, he had worked on a Clinical Scholars program and academic community health plans and had directed the Commonwealth Fund–Harvard University Press Book Program. "Frank Karel and I were both recruited to work for Commonwealth and began work on the same day in 1968," recalls Annie Lea Shuster, who began as Keenan's assistant at Commonwealth and later became a program officer at the Robert Wood Johnson Foundation. "Much of the thinking for the early Robert Wood Johnson programs was done at Commonwealth. In fact, the three of us would sit around having lunch in New York, talking about health care ideas and about moving the foundation to Princeton. A few years later, we were all there together."

⟶ Beginnings

In December 1971, the Robert Wood Johnson Foundation officially opened its doors in a modest Victorian house in New
Brunswick, New Jersey, with $1.2 billion in assets and the con-
gressional requirement to spend $45 million in grants by the end of
1972. Gustav Lienhard, who had resigned as president of Johnson
& Johnson on April 1, 1971, to become president and treasurer
of the new foundation, was a crusty, no-nonsense businessman
who announced his belief in "productive philanthropy."[3] David
Rogers, formerly dean of the Johns Hopkins University School
of Medicine, was named president as of January 1, 1972, while
Lienhard became its full-time Board chairman. Neither had ever
worked for a foundation, much less one of the largest philanthropic institutions in the United States—second only to the
Ford Foundation. Together, however, they assembled a remarkable team of health care experts that immediately forged new
directions in the foundation world.

Keenan joined the Robert Wood Johnson Foundation as a
senior executive associate in March 1972 (he was promoted to vice
president later that year), based on the strong recommendation
of Margaret Mahoney, who had been hired at the same time
from the Carnegie Corporation to be a vice president at Robert
Wood Johnson. ("As I remember it, Margaret said that she
wouldn't come unless I went, and I wouldn't go unless she
went," Keenan says. "So, happily, we went together.") Mahoney
and Keenan were joined by Robert Blendon, who had worked
with Rogers at Johns Hopkins and who is currently a professor
of health policy at Harvard's School of Public Health, and Walsh
McDermott, a physician and former chairman of the Department
of Public Health at Cornell University Medical College. This
quartet became Rogers's programmatic advisory group.

Because the staff was small at the beginning (twenty-one
people are listed in the 1972 Annual Report), ideas were shared
freely, and Rogers's style of leadership was casual. "We moved

to the Forrestal campus at Princeton University soon after the Foundation was formed," recalls Ruby Hearn, who joined Robert Wood Johnson in 1976 as a program officer and retired in 2001 as senior vice president. "We were upstairs in the Forrestal Center, the same building as a linear accelerator. Almost every day, the entire staff, including Dr. Rogers, would have lunch around a common table. In that atmosphere, Terry Keenan was most effective because he could share his ideas quietly. Because of Terry's gentle manner, he was at risk of being underestimated in a larger forum. In that small group, we listened and learned. A lot of the ideas that became very important to the Foundation were originally suggested and nurtured by Terry. He was sort of the progenitor of many of the most significant programs we have ever done."[4]

Terry was deliberately unimposing. He used to dress almost every day in a white shirt, tie, slacks, and a wonderful tan windbreaker jacket that he would hang on a coat rack. He rarely wore a formal sport coat or a suit. He'd be at his desk, which was always piled high with papers, and start each day with a fresh yellow-lined pad and a half dozen freshly sharpened number-two pencils. He looked like how you might imagine one of the editors at *The New York Times*. He was a wordsmith and always found the right phrase, whether he was writing a presentation to the Board or a memo to a colleague. Perhaps the most significant memory of Terry I have is that no matter how busy he was, he always made time to talk with a colleague.

—Alfred Sadler, former Robert Wood Johnson Foundation assistant vice president

Although it would be unfair to attribute specific programs solely to any individual in a collective effort such as the Robert Wood Johnson Foundation in its early years, many of the fifty-seven grants listed in the 1972 Annual Report clearly reflect Keenan's career-long areas of passionate concern. For example, the largest grant authorization to a single institution in that first year, $5 million, went to Meharry Medical College in Nashville, Tennessee, to enlarge its primary care teaching facilities. At that time, Meharry graduated half of the nation's practicing African American physicians and 80 percent of those practicing in the thirteen Southern states. Margaret Mahoney's Clinical Scholars Program to train young physicians for leadership roles, which she had brought to Robert Wood Johnson from the Carnegie and Commonwealth foundations, received a $5.9 million grant. This is a program that Keenan had enthusiastically championed and worked on closely with Mahoney before they both joined the Robert Wood Johnson Foundation. A grant of $4 million for dental student aid again reflected Keenan's career emphasis on the need for greater access to dental health care.

Several smaller grants suggest programmatic areas that would later flourish under Keenan's care: a program at the University of California, Davis, to train rural nurse practitioners; a health care system study in Montgomery, Alabama; a network of rural health clinics near Provo, Utah; a summer study program in Newark, New Jersey, to prepare minority students to enter the health professions; and a grant to the Foundation Center for data collection and analysis of foundations. All were from Keenan's first Robert Wood Johnson portfolio.

Moving Ideas into the Mainstream

On the north bank of the Yukon River, about 470 miles northwest of Anchorage, Alaska, there is a remote fishing settlement, an enclave accessible only by dogsled and snowmobile in the winter, bush plane and small boats after the thaw.

At the hub of this village, just below the Arctic Circle, is a very modest health center. It is staffed by nine Yupik Inuits, who have been trained as community health aides. They speak halting English as a second language, but beam with pride as they describe the eighteen-week training program that transformed their lives and brought medical care to their frontier town.

Terry Keenan funded that training program in 1975. When I visited Mountain Village, Alaska, last week, I found that the model had been replicated among the frontier settlements that dot the Alaskan tundra. Moving an idea from the margins to the mainstream ... that's Terry's forte. Terry also heralded nurse home visiting long before it was common. And there is no more genteel but dogged champion of nursing, midlevel professionals, training around domestic violence, services for the disabled, mobilizing volunteers for service, dental scholars, health care in public housing, minority student enrichment, early childhood literacy, parenting, and—of course—family centers.

—Judith Stavisky, Robert Wood Johnson Foundation senior program officer

"Terry was originally brought into Robert Wood Johnson for internal management purposes rather than programmatic ideas," recalls former Foundation vice president Robert Blendon.

After all, he and Margaret Mahoney were the only ones with much real foundation experience. However, it very quickly became apparent that he had lots of valuable ideas about the role of foundations in general and about particular programs in health care. He held the strong view that a large foundation like ours could help to develop a network of small or medium-size foundations to share information; this eventually led to the formation of Grantmakers In Health. He also saw that funding at the community level was more effective when shared with other partners, which led to our Local Initiative Funding Partners Program. He perceived very early that many of the problems of health care had to do with shortages of nurses, the quality of nurse training, and the lack of leadership in the field. He made a very strong case for the value of faith-based health care programs, and argued that the Foundation should not be exclusively secular in its funding. He brought our attention to programs for dental health care, school-based adolescent health care, and other areas. But if I had to name Terry's greatest contribution to Robert Wood Johnson, it would be his relentless insistence that we never forget those vulnerable populations—elderly, disabled, children, minorities—who need health care in the inner cities and, most especially, all those small towns across America.

An examination of the astonishing 942 grants championed and supervised by Keenan supports Blendon's judgment. The grants in this portfolio have been made to numerous small community organizations all over the United States. A few are for millions of dollars and a few are for less than $10,000; most are for less than $100,000—modest by Robert Wood Johnson Foundation standards. Although Keenan's emphasis upon community initiatives, interfaith caregiving, school-based clinics, nursing, primary care for vulnerable populations, dental training, and services for the disabled and elderly are well represented, his commitments range across virtually every aspect of health and health care.

—⟋⟍— Local Initiative Funding Partners Program

From the beginning of Keenan's foundation career, he focused on community health care programs—particularly in small communities—and he quickly saw the need for a major reorganization of community funding practices. At the Ford Foundation and the Commonwealth Fund, he observed that local programs often disappeared after an initial three-year grant period. The grantees rarely made provisions for continued financial support. "The issue isn't what you can do about it, it's what you have to do about it," Keenan has observed. "You have to work on it and think about it and try to find ways to solve it. If you don't solve the problem, you can at least move the capacity to solve the problem more precisely and more vigorously ahead."[5]

Keenan set about finding a solution to the community health care problem through just the kind of inquiry he mentions. Rather than staying secure in the ivory tower of foundation offices, Keenan embarked on fact-finding missions in the field while simultaneously pursuing ways to partner with local philanthropic organizations. A trip to Texas in the late 1970s gave him a new insight into the problem. Journalist Irene Wielawski relates, "Keenan vividly remembers a trip to Texas, in which he called on foundations from one end of the state to the other trying to get them interested in financing a start-up health clinic in an abandoned church in San Antonio... Keenan essentially acted as their ambassador."[6]

He failed in that effort. He was viewed as the voice of a big Yankee foundation that was not only meddling but also arrogant. Quite reasonably, local philanthropies wanted to know why, if the Robert Wood Johnson Foundation thought this health clinic was such a good idea, it didn't provide some funding. Chastened by his experience in Texas, Keenan realized that "it would be easier to get a favorable reception if I had some money to put on the table."

His earlier experimentation with funneling money into grassroots programs had resulted in the first community-based program of the Foundation, the Community Care Funding Partners Program, in the early 1980s. This program was characterized by its process: localized grant applications for school-based clinics and other primary care units had to satisfy a Foundation requirement for dollar-for-dollar matching funds from a local partnering funder. The idea was that the partnering institution would stay on and even help to gather additional funding after the Robert Wood Johnson Foundation's initial support ended. Frank Karel, former vice president of communications at the Foundation, called Keenan's idea "a stroke of genius," and noted, "No big foundation had ever done anything like this."

"I accompanied him on a site visit to Hazlehurst, Georgia, a small mill town in a rural community south of Macon," Peter Goodwin, the Foundation's vice president for national program affairs, recalls.

> I can't remember how long it took us to get there, but it seemed like forever. He had been there before, and they knew he was coming to

discuss their plans for a community health center that he had funded through the Foundation. I thought we were meeting with two or three people. But when we rolled into town, you would have thought the president of the United States was arriving. I'd never in my life seen such a spectacle. The whole town of about 350 people rolled out the red carpet for us. They literally closed down the town and took us to their country club, where the sheriff, who was attending, looked the other way about the local blue laws and joined in the toast to Terry Keenan. We were both embarrassed by this display of appreciation, but it was the most tangible evidence I've ever had that we are doing the right thing at the Foundation.

The full-scale Local Initiative Funding Partners program did not emerge until 1987, with a mandate to expand the scope of the Community Care Funding Partners program beyond funding for local clinics. The new entity gave considerable power to local philanthropies in selecting projects that they believed were deserving of support. Not surprisingly, many of the program's first grants dealt with such pressing but controversial social problems as child sex abuse, drug abuse, teen pregnancy, and HIV infection. At the center of the new program lay Keenan's sense of social responsibility. Musing on a foundation's raison d'être, he later remarked, "I think that foundations working with other entities at the local, state, but also the national level can use their funds not only for convening but for looking at issues and understanding problems. If you go back to what foundation philanthropy represents in our society, it really is the principal source of private development capital investing in social purposes."[7]

Despite giving local voices a hearing, however, there were internal problems with the plan at the Foundation. According to Irene Wielawski, "It stood out as a radical departure from the status quo, and discomfort within the staff was palpable."[8] In response to internal pressures as well as a curtailment of grantmaking in general, the program was shut down in 1989, at the end of its second round of funding.

But Keenan did not give up; he adopted a ruminative position instead. Pauline Seitz, current director of the Local Initiative Funding Partners program, recalls, "Terry never hesitated to just roll over, pretending he was dead... It was sort of a turtle technique that Terry had. He would just get bombarded and critiqued from all sides, and he'd sort of go into his shell ... and when nobody was looking he'd just crawl out very slowly and proceed back on course, and he'd inevitably get across the finish line."

> I had just concluded a wonderful job interview with Terry for a job as program officer for the Local Initiative Funding Partners program in August of 1987 and we were waiting for my next interviewer to be available. He looked out of his office, across the atrium to the other offices in the building and seemed to be lost in thought for a moment. He turned to me and said, "You know, working here isn't for everybody. The Foundation is sort of like the Wizard of Oz, and you have to stay behind the curtain. You have to understand that the most significant work of the organization is done by the grantees. We are simply the agents of their success, and they deserve the credit. If you have a need for direct recognition, it can be a very frustrating environment, because everything that happens here takes place behind the mask of that Wizard called the Robert Wood Johnson Foundation."
>
> —Pauline Seitz, director of the Local Initiative Funding Partners program

Steven Schroeder recalls that when he became president of the Robert Wood Johnson Foundation, in 1990, he felt an almost immediate kinship with Keenan. "One of the first things I did when I moved into the Foundation offices was to place on my desk a quotation sent to me by my friend, John Kenneth Galbraith," Schroeder says. "It reads, 'Nothing so gives the illusion of intelligence as a personal association with large sums of money.' Terry liked that quote, and he helped me to guard against

Foundation arrogance by his example and by the occasional quiet comment."

Before his appointment, Schroeder candidly informed the Board of the Robert Wood Johnson Foundation that he intended to lead the Foundation in a more active role to combat the social roots of health care problems in America. One of his first acts was to reinstate the Local Initiative Funding Partners program. "Terry's program was central to how I thought the Foundation should operate," Schroeder recalls. "It permitted us to have an ear to the ground all throughout the country; to work through others; to honor those others; to be a senior but equal partner; and to respect people. It is a great grassroots program." As Schroeder recalls, there was still internal resistance when he revived the program, and Keenan was "not a glamorous salesman, but he was a tenacious salesman. Ultimately, I think all of our staff became very proud of that program."[9]

In a memorandum of October 24, 1990, to Schroeder, Keenan suggested some new rules to address a problem that faced the Local Initiative program. The Foundation had been requiring its local foundation partners to guarantee that matching funds would be made available, even before the Foundation had itself agreed to fund a project. This created resentments since, as Irene Wielawski has written, "Qualifying for the Foundation match translated into months of effort, including personal and public advocacy. . . The design flaw was potentially fatal to the Foundation's goal of genuine partnership with communities."[10] Keenan recommended that the Foundation drop the controversial requirement that partner-funders guarantee matching funds before the Robert Wood Johnson Foundation made a commitment—a recommendation that was accepted. Today, local funders are simply asked for a statement of intention instead of a guarantee of matching funds.

"The Local Initiative Funding Partners Program was an outstanding contribution," Schroeder points out. "Terry nurtured it at a time when it wasn't that popular. Now it is part of the Foundation's DNA."

—⚬— Interfaith Caregiving

Perhaps no other program exemplifies Terry Keenan's strong sense of coalition building better than the Foundation's interfaith partnership efforts. Keenan is a man of strong spiritual beliefs, and he keeps them private. From his earliest days at the Foundation, Keenan saw the value of partnering with hospitals, community medical centers, and local organizations that were faith-based. Understandably, there was considerable opposition within the Foundation to the appearance of financing religious institutions. After a decade of making small grants, the Foundation committed to a major initiative in 1983 with a $2.3 million grant to the fledgling Interfaith Volunteer Caregivers Program. The funding would provide three-year grants of $50,000 a year to fifteen churches, synagogues, and other houses of worship in fifteen communities around the country to set up coalitions where members of their different faith communities would provide care—such as transportation to doctors' offices, shopping, and companionship—to chronically ill people.

The Interfaith Caregivers Program was clearly a test of Keenan's conviction that a health services foundation should help tackle day-to-day issues of chronic care along with more traditional health services—and could do so by fostering partnerships of religious organizations. He recognized that "It should be possible to foster common purpose among institutions with similar missions—service to youth, for example—without loss of individual identity."[11] He identified this sense of common purpose in the general call to service that is part of the religious doctrine of many faiths. But he realized that within the well-intentioned efforts of most churches or synagogues lay the possibility of redundancy of effort. If the Foundation could foster interfaith programs sharing resources and person power, the crying need for volunteer caregiving could be harnessed and focused.

The initial announcement of the program was met by more than a thousand letters of intent from organizations all over the country. In response, the Foundation increased the number of sites from ten to twenty-five. Under the aegis of Kenneth Johnson, an internist at Kingston Hospital in Kingston, New York, and director of its health services research center, a demonstration program was launched with twenty-five interfaith coalitions. Johnson had worked closely with several previous Foundation programs. The money supported a paid director to coordinate and direct the volunteer efforts of these religious organizations. The rationale for paid directors stemmed from the idea that a paid staff person could better structure the enterprise, organize volunteers, and continually revise and adapt the plan for caregiving than a council of representatives, who might meet only sporadically. Many of the locations and other auxiliary supplies were provided by member denominations. Johnson observed, "Interfaith volunteer caregiver programs fill gaps in the long-term care system."[12]

The fact that ten years later, twenty of the initial twenty-five interfaith groups were still in existence testified not only to the need but also to the viability of these groups working together. Such was the positive response that in 1993 the Foundation invited interfaith caregiving organizations to submit applications for a new program, called Faith in Action, that replicated and expanded the concept. The program's supporters envisioned making enough grants so that eventually an interfaith coalition could exist in almost every corner of the United States.[13]

Each location needed to exhibit certain features, including:

- An authentic interfaith or ecumenical governance, involving a broad spectrum of faiths and denominations working together
- An average number of fifty volunteers serving fifty persons during the first twelve months of the program

- Volunteer caregiving that was direct, person-to-person, and hands-on, and that provided multiple kinds of assistance rather than a single service

Technical assistance was provided by twelve federation-sponsored regional facilitators, who were to help the coalitions make applications, build the coalitions, and secure matching funds and other administrative services.

Under the second round of funding for Faith in Action, 1,091 interfaith coalitions received Foundation support. In July 1998, when the last of the second-round grants had been awarded, nearly 60,000 people were volunteering their services under Faith in Action, or an average of fifty-seven volunteers per site.

In September 1999, the Foundation approved a third generation of the Faith in Action program. The retooled program, which sought to distribute $100 million to two thousand new faith-based coalitions over a seven-year period, was intended to expand its reach by coordinating with heretofore untraditional organizations such as the National Council of La Raza and the Islamic Society of North America. Features included grants of $35,000 per site, more technical support, and a new computer network that links coalitions and pools a variety of online resources.

In 2004, the Foundation decided to make final funding authorization to the program and to concentrate its resources on other initiatives. Nonetheless, Faith in Action is considered by many as a signature program of the Foundation. The credit, former Foundation vice president Paul Jellinek says, goes to Terry Keenan: "He was at the forefront of the interfaith caregiving movement, which started with a small demonstration program that Terry pushed through the Foundation back in 1983. The Robert Wood Johnson Foundation has now supported 1,100 of these coalitions around the country. It all goes back to Terry and his feelings about impact and scale."

—∿— Nurses' Training; Physician's Assistants; Emergency Medical Services

"Nurturing, caring, healing—that's what drives nursing, that caring sense," Keenan says. "It is really the ethos of the profession. I am very proud that the Foundation has taken a leadership role in the development of nursing, expanding the content of nursing, building up the education of nurses, and supporting the concept of the nurse practitioner. One of my first projects at the Foundation was to support nursing schools, particularly at the graduate level. To my amazement, a lot of people—including some of the deans of these schools—disagreed with that idea [graduate-level nurse practitioners]."

"It is strange to recall how controversial all the issues around nurses and nurse practitioners were at the beginning," says Ruby Hearn, former Robert Wood Johnson Foundation senior vice president. "Doctors were upset about the financial aspects of their roles and what medical functions nurses might be authorized to perform. Terry was particularly supportive of clinics run by freestanding nurse practitioners, and that was extremely controversial. Of course, today, the expanded role of nurses and nurse practitioners is considered an absolutely necessary part of the medical establishment."

As with so many of Keenan's ideas, his concepts about nursing—including an expanded role for nurses, specialized medical training for nurses and physician's assistants, restructuring of hospital nursing care, use of emergency registered nurses in remote rural areas, and clinics headed by nurse practitioners—were considered revolutionary in the 1970s.[14] "My brother Blair and I first met Terry Keenan in the summer of 1970 at the Commonwealth Fund, in that beautiful old building of theirs on the corner of 75th Street and Central Park," recalls Alfred Sadler, a former Robert Wood Johnson Foundation assistant vice president. "The Fund had just granted $2 million for a very imaginative program in emergency medicine and trauma management under the direction of Jack Cole, who was chairman of surgery at the Yale School of Medicine."[15] Blair and Alfred Sadler, identical twins, were hired to run this program, and they quickly convinced Cole that Yale should sponsor a program for physician's assistants in emergency care that was similar to the pioneering Duke University Physician Assistant program in general medicine under Eugene Stead.

"During our three years at Yale, Fred and I stayed in close communication with Terry at Commonwealth and Maggie Mahoney at Carnegie," says Blair Sadler, who is also a former Robert Wood Johnson Foundation assistant vice president. "In fact, they supported us and encouraged us to write *The Physician's Assistant—Today and Tomorrow* (Yale University Press, 1972) with a colleague at Yale, Ann Bliss. This was a summary of the work we had done and of the developments in the field at that point. To give you an illustration of how closely we worked together, that book is dedicated to Terry and Maggie."

In 1973, David Rogers, then the president of the Robert Wood Johnson Foundation, came to Yale to give a speech and met the Sadlers. After that meeting and some discussions with Keenan and Mahoney, who were already at the Robert Wood Johnson Foundation, Rogers invited the Sadlers to join the Foundation and to take their successful Yale Emergency Medical Services program nationwide. "We couldn't believe the collegial atmosphere at the Foundation headquarters in Princeton," Blair Sadler recalls. "The entire staff would sit around a lunch table and dream about how to solve the health care problems of the United States. Terry never dominated these casual meetings, but when he spoke everyone listened carefully, because he always had insights and ideas that were based on his experiences in the field. He was passionate about the need for training and utilizing physician assistants and nurse practitioners."

"From those early days to the present, Terry Keenan's achievements have been remarkable," Alfred Sadler says. "But more than that, his influence, his personality, and his thinking about grantmaking have been hugely influential in the whole world of philanthropy, especially in medical and health care foundations. His humanistic approach, his willingness to take risks, or even fail, and his concern that foundations have to look to the future—Terry has changed foundation culture for the better by his example."

Although Keenan has always credited many Robert Wood Johnson Foundation colleagues for their important contributions—including Margaret Mahoney, the Sadlers, Linda Aiken, Ruby Hearn, and Nancy Kaufman—there is no doubt that he took the initiative in advancing multiple changes in the world of nursing. "Terry was very committed to school-based clinics when I arrived at the Foundation in 1972," recalls Edward Robbins, former director of the office of proposal management at the Foundation. "The area was controversial for many reasons. First, it was a new area for the Foundation, which had been accustomed to working with hospitals and universities. Second, religious and political organizations objected to nurses providing birth control information to adolescents. And, third, doctors were uncomfortable with the expanded diagnostic role nurses were playing in these schools. Quite frankly, in many cases, the nurses were taking more initiative about the children's health care than the parents were."

Some of the grants in Keenan's 1972 portfolio included funding for a nurse practitioner program for rural areas that was supervised by the new Department of Family Practice at the University of California, Davis, and training for nurse practitioners at the Utah Valley Hospital in Provo. Keenan championed grants to the Tuskegee Institute in Alabama in 1973 and 1974 to utilize teams of nurse practitioners working from a mobile van to make an initial assessment of the health needs of families in a three-county area of Alabama; in 1974, he convinced the Foundation to provide funding for Kentucky's Frontier Nursing Service to develop a curriculum for training of family nurse practitioners; and in that same year he recommended a grant to

Adelphi University in Garden City, New York, to study the role of nurses in primary care. By 1978, the Foundation, based on Keenan's recommendations, had funded more than a dozen nurse and physician's assistant training programs around the country. These included the Program to Equip Emergency Nurses with Primary Care Skills to train emergency room nurses from small regional hospitals in six university-affiliated hospitals, and the School Health Services Program, which brought nurse practitioners to 150,000 children of low-income parents in thirty-six urban elementary schools, and which was the first of a number of Foundation-funded school-based health programs.

A lot of people at foundations are basically academics. They don't like to get their hands dirty or to come out of the ivory tower. Well, Terry was just the opposite. For example, in 1988, he heard about a program for poor children in Chicago called Project Beethoven. As always, he didn't just pick up the telephone. He got on the plane to Chicago. So here is Terry, by this time in his career an older gentleman and a little frail from just having had cardiac bypass surgery, going into the worst neighborhood in the South Side of Chicago. It was extremely rough at the time. Mothers were afraid to allow their children to play on the playgrounds. There was crack cocaine addiction and people shooting at each other every day. You could get killed just getting out of a taxicab in this neighborhood. Here comes gray-haired Terry, all by himself, walking down the block, trying to find the right address. People from the project looked out of a second-story window and saw him picking his way over piles of trash. They ran down the stairs to get him.

His hosts told me that they were horrified when he arrived alone. But he put them at ease. He sat down with them and listened to their problems. He went into the classrooms and met the children. Then he came back to the Foundation and wrote a million-dollar grant to build a health clinic and to develop a coordinated plan to link the public health nursing, social services, and educational services for the children. From there, Terry went on to create a whole child development initiative for the country. He brought in other foundations and showed them how to replicate this model of providing sanctuaries for children within very bad neighborhoods. He basically revolutionized the field, and today there are hundreds of child development centers all over the country based on the ideas he initiated at Beethoven.

—Nancy Kaufman, former vice president at the Robert Wood Johnson Foundation

The Foundation has continued to support the field of nursing, including the $7 million Teaching Nursing Home Program, the $11 million Clinical Nurse Scholars Program, the $17 million program for Strengthening Hospital Nursing, the $29.7 million Executive Nurse Fellows Program, and the $1.8 million Transforming Care at the Bedside Program. Nurse practitioners and physician assistants have become a recognized part of America's health care system. The Foundation has given more than $140 million to nursing programs, and continues its strong commitment to the field.[16]

—⋙— Grantmakers In Health

Almost from the moment Terry Keenan arrived at the Foundation, he began networking with other foundations. He shared information about the activities of the Robert Wood Johnson Foundation and, in many cases, attempted to coordinate funding of programs. There were a limited number of philanthropies in the United States that were working on health issues, and Keenan was aware that they never sat down at a table together to discuss common problems or to learn from one another. For more than a decade, he acted as a one-man communications center among the health care foundations, until he was able to create a national organization called Grantmakers In Health in 1982.

Grantmakers In Health now brings together some 330 foundations and corporate grantmaking organizations in a regular series of meetings, workshops, issue-focused forums, and publications about health and health care issues. Since 1998, it also has operated the Resource Center on Health Philanthropy, which collects data from health philanthropies and identifies trends in the field. As a tribute to his importance in the field, the Terrance Keenan Leadership Award in Health Philanthropy is presented by Grantmakers In Health every year to an outstanding individual in the field. "We feel that this award recognizes Mr. Keenan's importance in health philanthropy, and regularly reminds us of his values and spirit," says Lauren LeRoy, president and chief executive officer of Grantmakers In Health.

—⁓— An Appreciation

"Terry's heartfelt compassion for the most vulnerable in our society came across in the way he approached philanthropy," Risa Lavizzo-Mourey, president and CEO of the Foundation, said in a speech honoring Keenan last year. "When Terry joined the Robert Wood Johnson Foundation, foundations in general were not terribly active; they did not have a mission and a program for change. In fact, philanthropy was considered suspect by many people who believed wealthy individuals were establishing foundations to use as tax write-offs. Terry helped change both the reality and the perception of foundations." In that same speech, she said, "Describing someone as a 'legend' may seem excessive. But in the case of Terrance Keenan, the term is entirely appropriate."

Notes

1. Keenan, T. *The Promise at Hand*. Princeton, NJ: Robert Wood Johnson Foundation Publications, 1992. Unpublished revised manuscript, 2003.
2. Jellinek, P. Speech at Grantmakers In Health, Terrance Keenan Award luncheon, March 2, 2000, Miami.

3. Pace University website. Gustav O. Lienhard biography, http://webpage.pace.edu/mweigold/lienhardbio.html.
4. Interview with Ruby Hearn, November 20, 2004.
5. Keenan, T. Speech at Grantmakers In Health Awards ceremonies, March 2, 2000, Miami.
6. Wielawski, I. M. "The Local Initiative Funding Partners Program." *To Improve Health and Health Care 2000: The Robert Wood Johnson Foundation Anthology*. San Francisco: Jossey-Bass, 1999.
7. Keenan, T. Grantmakers In Health Awards ceremonies, 2000.
8. Wielawski, p. 162.
9. Ibid.
10. Ibid.
11. Keenan, T. Preface. Reflections on Grantmaking, http://www.rwjf.org/library/reflect7.htm.
12. Faith in Action National Program Report, updated April 2004, http://www.rwjf.org/reports/nreports/faithinaction.htm.
13. Jellinek, P., Gibbs Appel, T., and Keenan, T. "Faith in Action." *To Improve Health and Health Care 1998–1999: The Robert Wood Johnson Foundation Anthology*. San Francisco: Jossey-Bass, 1998.
14. Keenan, T. "Support of Nurse Practitioners and Physician Assistants." *To Improve Health and Health Care 1998–1999: The Robert Wood Johnson Foundation Anthology*. San Francisco: Jossey-Bass, 1998.
15. Diehl, D. "The Emergency Medical Services Program." *To Improve Health and Health Care 1998–1999: The Robert Wood Johnson Foundation Anthology*. San Francisco: Jossey-Bass, 1998.
16. Newbergh, C. "The Robert Wood Johnson Foundation's Commitment to Nursing." *To Improve Health and Health Care: The Robert Wood Johnson Foundation Anthology*, Vol. VIII. San Francisco: Jossey-Bass, 2005.

CHAPTER 4

The Five Cs

Risa Lavizzo-Mourey

Editors' Introduction

The Robert Wood Johnson Foundation has always considered itself a "strategic" philanthropy, that is, one whose goal is to move public policy in ways that will improve the nation's health. Employing this approach, the Foundation is able to leverage the effect of its relatively limited resources and to have greater impact than it would by, say, making a series of grants to charitable organizations.

In his first *Annual Report* as the Foundation's president, David Rogers articulated the philosophy, writing that the Foundation sought to bring about "worthwhile social change" and that "we are limiting our work to a few selected areas because history suggests that meaningful change is brought about only when there is a critical mass of people or institutions working on the solution of a particular problem." Nearly twenty years later, in *his* first annual report, Steven Schroeder touched upon the same issue, noting, "If the Foundation is to have any impact on the way this nation delivers its health care, it must be forever watchful that its mission, goals and strategies are tightly focused and relevant."

A strategic approach implies not only focusing on a limited number of issues but also bringing to bear all of the tools available to philanthropy. It means, as Schroeder wrote in the 1990 *Annual Report*, "a shift ... toward integrated approaches that encompass the full range of philanthropic interventions." Yet even with the Foundation's long history of attempting to effect social change and employing a variety of interventions to do so, the program staff, in the early 2000s, saw its role primarily as grantmakers, rather than change makers.

Early in her presidency, Risa Lavizzo-Mourey recognized the disconnect between a foundation endeavoring to change society and a staff viewing itself simply as a dispenser of money. This prompted her to examine the various ways in which foundations, and the Robert Wood Johnson Foundation in particular, could influence public policy and led her to write "the five Cs." First presented to the Board in 2005, the five Cs captures what the Foundation has done and can do to bring about social change. Reprinted as a foreword to Volume IX of the *Robert Wood Johnson Foundation Anthology*, the piece should have resonance for the field of philanthropy as a whole.*

---

* Because this was written as a foreword to Volume IX of the *Anthology*, the references to chapters in the reprint refer to chapters in that volume, not the current one.

In keeping our promise to improve the health and health care of all Americans, the Robert Wood Johnson Foundation has developed an Impact Framework that sets long-, medium-, and short-term objectives for each of our priority areas.[1] Over the past few years, we have become increasingly sophisticated about using all of our resources to achieve these objectives. Although writing checks may be central to our work, we have many other tools at our disposal. Among them are what I call "the five Cs" of effective philanthropy, and the way we employ them can be seen throughout this volume of *The Robert Wood Johnson Foundation Anthology*. The five Cs are:

- *Communicating*. The Foundation has always placed a high value on sharing the results of our work and that of our grantees.[2] Historically, we have emphasized speaking through our grantees. Now we are trying to speak with our grantees, to be more open in our communications about our own objectives, and to ensure that different audiences get the information they need in a form that they can use and from a source they can trust. The chapter by Susan Krutt and David Morse (Chapter 9) illustrates the ways in which the Foundation fosters transparency and public accountability. It is complemented by the discussion of Cover the Uninsured Week, a series of communications campaigns designed to keep the uninsured in the public's consciousness, in Robert Rosenblatt's chapter (Chapter 3) on the Foundation's efforts to promote health insurance coverage.

- *Convening*. The Robert Wood Johnson Foundation has used its prestige and its influence to bring together people who might not ordinarily be in the same room. Perhaps the best recent example is our convening of what we call the "strange bedfellows," discussed in Chapter 3, which brought together health insurance experts with differing positions to see whether they could agree on an approach to covering the uninsured. Although they do not agree on a single approach, the strange bedfellows do agree on some general principles and are continuing to explore options to achieve those principles. On a local scale, under the Free to Grow program, examined by Irene Wielawski in Chapter 1, community leaders working with the Head Start program were able to mobilize residents with varied interests who were all concerned about drug and alcohol abuse by young people in their community.

■ *Coordinating*. Although it takes time, requires considerable interpersonal skills, and too often is unrewarded, coordination among multiple stakeholders, especially other funders, is essential. A deft touch is required, and no one has had a defter touch than legendary grantmaker Terrance Keenan, whom we honor in Chapter 8. In fostering the growth of nurse practitioners and physician assistants, the Foundation, through Keenan, was able to work with and coordinate the efforts of the federal government, academic medical centers, and the nursing profession, among others. As noted by the chapter's author, Digby Diehl, the Foundation, under Keenan's tutelage, developed the Local Initiative Funding Partners program, in which the Robert Wood Johnson Foundation collaborates with local foundations in funding projects that they have identified. Students Run LA, described by Paul Brodeur in Chapter 7, is a prime example of an effective project funded through the Local Initiative Funding Partners program.

■ *Connecting*. Individual grants become more powerful when one grant builds on another and when the lessons from one project inform others. Continuity and connectivity are often the hallmarks of a well-executed strategy. One of the roles the Foundation plays is connecting the dots—helping grantees see how their own work fits into a larger scheme to meet bigger objectives. In their chapter on healthy aging (Chapter 2), Robin Mockenhaupt, Jane Isaacs Lowe, and Geralyn Graf Magan demonstrate how a group of seemingly disparate grants are in reality elements in a larger strategy, or series of strategies, to improve the health and well-being of older Americans. Similarly, in Chapter 6, Victor Capoccia discusses the evolution of the Foundation's approach to combating drug and alcohol addiction and how individual grants reflect and advance the Foundation's strategies.

- *Counting*. Monitoring progress by using rigorous and appropriately timed indicators is critical to knowing whether change is taking place. This has long been a hallmark of the Robert Wood Johnson Foundation. Chapters in earlier volumes of the *Anthology* have discussed the Foundation's research and evaluation efforts and the work of grantees such as the Center for Studying Health System Change.[3] In this volume, Marsha Gold and her colleagues Justin White and Erin Fries Taylor at Mathematica Policy Research write about their evaluation of the Medicaid Managed Care Program. The chapter (Chapter 5) illustrates not only the importance of timely assessments but also their value in providing an empirical basis for shifting the emphasis of a program.

The use of the five Cs—combined with a sixth C, cash—can be powerful indeed. Perhaps the best example of the Foundation's using the Cs strategically is its work to reduce smoking between 1990 and the present.[4] The challenge for the Robert Wood Johnson Foundation is to employ all the tools available to it aggressively and purposefully. If we do so, we greatly increase our potential impact and the likelihood of achieving long-lasting returns in health and well-being.

Notes

1. See the Foundation's website for a listing of the Foundation's portfolios and teams (www.rwjf.org).
2. Karel, F. "'Getting the Word Out': A Foundation Memoir and Personal Journey." *To Improve Health and Health Care 2001: The Robert Wood Johnson Foundation Anthology*. San Francisco: Jossey-Bass, 2001.
3. Knickman, J. "Research as a Foundation Strategy." *To Improve Health and Health Care 2000: The Robert Wood Johnson Foundation Anthology*. San Francisco: Jossey-Bass, 1999. Newbergh, C. "The Health Tracking Initiative." *To Improve Health and Health Care: The Robert Wood Johnson Foundation Anthology*, Vol. VI. San Francisco: Jossey-Bass, 2003.
4. Isaacs, S. L. and Knickman, J. R. "Field Building: Lessons from The Robert Wood Johnson Foundation Anthology Series." *Health Affairs*, 2005, *24*(4), 1161–1165.

CHAPTER 5

The Robert Wood Johnson Foundation's Approach to Evaluation

James R. Knickman and Kelly A. Hunt

Editors' Introduction

A hallmark of the Robert Wood Johnson Foundation is its commitment to evaluation. In its second year, 1973, the Foundation commissioned evaluations of two programs it had funded the previous year—Emergency Medical Systems and Aid for Students in Medicine and Osteopathy.

In this chapter, reprinted from Volume XI of the *Anthology*, James Knickman, the Foundation's vice president for research and evaluation at the time, and Kelly Hunt, then a Foundation research and evaluation officer, describe four tiers of evaluation—measuring the impact of specific programs; tracking the impact of a portfolio of programs; assessing organizational effectiveness; and informing the public with Program Results Reports and the *Anthology*. Since the publication of the chapter, the Foundation's approach has evolved, and it has added to the tiers of evaluation two new methods to measure the results of its work.

The first has to do with methodology. The Foundation is now using the "systematic screening and assessment method" to identify innovations that are worth evaluating and are likely to have impact.[1] This approach identifies promising interventions that warrant being evaluated and conducts assessments to determine whether the interventions can be evaluated, after which an expert panel reviews and ranks the interventions for their potential impact. This process allows the Foundation to identify promising innovations for replication, thus saving money and speeding up their adoption. Currently, this is being used to assess innovations in childhood obesity, access to dental care, and primary care. In addition, the Foundation is beginning to use social network analysis—a sociological technique to understand the relationships and interactions among individuals and organizations—to evaluate the influence of the Foundation, its grantees, and the research it supports.

The second method is an in-depth analysis of a portfolio of related programs that have been completed. This is called the retrospectives series.[2] Each retrospective is designed to answer four questions:

- Which programs worked and which didn't?
- What was the impact of the portfolio?
- Were the results greater than the sum of the parts?
- What are the grantmaking lessons from the body of work?

Probably the most important lesson to emerge from the retrospectives so far is that the Foundation is most likely to reach its strategic goals when it develops and implements programs that work together synergistically.

These retrospectives have led to the Foundation's conducting midcourse reviews on all areas of its work. Although the midcourse reviews are not as thorough as the retrospectives, they have played an important part in refining the Foundation's strategies.

A decade and half after the Foundation was founded as a national philanthropy, the sociologist Howard Freeman wrote that "the Foundation's commitment to evaluation is one of the distinctive features of its overall program."[3] Today, after forty years as a national philanthropy, evaluation remains a distinctive feature, and it pervades all aspects of the Foundation's work.

Notes

1. Leviton, L. C., Kettel Khan, L., and Dawkins, N. (eds.). "The Systematic Screening and Assessment Method: Finding Innovations Worth Evaluating." *New Directions in Evaluation*, No. 125 (Spring 2010).

2. Four Retrospectives are available at www.rwjf.org: Improving Care at the End of Life, The Tobacco Campaigns, Chronic Care Programs, and Reducing Harm from Alcohol and Drugs.

3. Freeman, H. E. *A Review of the Robert Wood Johnson's Evaluations of Its National Programs* (unpublished paper, 1987).

In philanthropy, as in business, the bottom line counts. But each sector measures the bottom line differently. Businesses can look to revenue, income, sales, earnings per share, and other quantitative indicators to measure performance. Foundations often work with less clear-cut indicators of impact. Sometimes they find it difficult to quantify the objective they wish to achieve. At other times it is difficult to know whether social change is due to the actions of a foundation or to other forces.

Over the past twenty years, the imperative to evaluate outcomes and assess effectiveness has become progressively important in philanthropy. Government leaders and others who watch philanthropy increasingly push for evidence that foundations use their resources wisely and actually contribute to addressing social problems. Boards of trustees at foundations have also become increasingly demanding when it comes to accountability and impact.

This imperative for evaluation is most characteristic among foundations that attempt to effect social change in active, coordinated ways. If a foundation chooses to focus on direct charity—funding services at homeless shelters, say, or supporting free medical care for the uninsured—the links between social contributions and the foundation's resources are generally considered self-evident. The impact of such contributions can be measured by the number of people served or by improvement in their health. When a foundation focuses on making grants that address a social problem, such as efforts to end homelessness or to bring about universal health insurance coverage, then it becomes more difficult to demonstrate a causal relationship between a foundation's investment and a change in the social environment.

The Robert Wood Johnson Foundation is generally regarded as a foundation that takes evaluation and performance assessment seriously. It has a staff of twelve professionals plus support staff members focused on evaluation, and it has been conducting evaluations of grants since its earliest days, in the 1970s.

—∿— Historical Roots

The idea of evaluating the effectiveness of grant programs came naturally to the early leaders of the Foundation. The board of directors consisted largely of recently retired Johnson & Johnson executives and others who had been colleagues of the founder. Accustomed to drug trials in which the effectiveness of a new pharmaceutical product is rigorously tested before being placed on the market, the board looked for comparable approaches to judging the impact of Foundation programs. Many of the Foundation's earliest investments were multisite demonstrations of new approaches to improving access to health care. Multiple states or communities or providers would be funded to try a specified strategy for, say, improving access. This type of grantmaking warranted investments in program evaluations to determine whether or not the new approach in fact had beneficial impacts. Given the interest of the Foundation in identifying ideas that could, if successful, serve as models, evaluation emerged as a central feature of its approach to grantmaking over the years.

Additionally, the 1970s, when the field of public policy analysis was emerging, were years of ferment in the area of social science research. It was natural to borrow the evaluation methods being used by the federal government to test new approaches to delivering services to low-income individuals ("social experiments"). In the 1970s, for example, the federal government financed a range of social experiments that tested new ideas in welfare reform, national health insurance models, and workforce training.

The emphasis on formal evaluations of large-scale programs continued through the 1980s, and it continues today for programs that test new ideas for improving health care or promoting the public's health. During the 1980s and 1990s, however, the Foundation's grantmaking approaches became more diversified as it funded research to understand health challenges such as the lack of insurance coverage; communications efforts to increase public awareness about a range of health problems and potential solutions to them; and wide-ranging programs to address health problems such as smoking. The board also applied pressure to broaden the approaches used by the Foundation to assess impact. Board members asked two types of questions: What are we learning from all of these grants? and How can we be sure that our grants are really making a difference in improving health or health care?

As a result, in the 1990s evaluation at the Foundation began to change in important ways. Instead of just asking whether a specific grant program was effective, the Foundation began looking at groups of grants that were meant to affect a specific health problem and assessing whether the grants as a group were effective in addressing it. It developed a family of evaluation tools focused on different aspects of impact. The Foundation currently uses a four-tiered approach to evaluation.

- The first tier attempts to understand the effectiveness of specific programs. Following its well-established pattern, the Foundation hires outside institutions to evaluate the results of its major grant initiatives.

- The second tier attempts to understand the impact of clusters of programs that focus on a particular goal or set of goals. In 2003, the Foundation developed an impact framework that sets short-, long-, and medium-range targets in specific program areas (such as health insurance coverage, childhood obesity, and public health).[1] Concurrently, it developed performance indicators to measure progress toward those targets.

- The third tier examines how the Foundation as an organization is doing, using a "scorecard" that is presented to the board annually. The scorecard incorporates the impact framework's performance indicators and commissions surveys to find out what grantees think of the Foundation, what experts think the Foundation's impact on health is, and what the staff considers to be the Foundation's strong and weak points.

- The fourth tier assesses the work of the Foundation in a less formal way and presents the results to a broad public. This collaborative program-evaluation-communications effort uses two vehicles: (1) grant results reports, in which the Foundation commissions writers to investigate specific grants and grant programs and write reports on them that appear on the Foundation's website, and (2) *To Improve Health and Health Care: The Robert Wood Johnson Foundation Anthology*, the book series published annually by Jossey-Bass. Both of these vehicles focus on disseminating what the Foundation has learned from various aspects of its grantmaking.

—᷈— Tier 1: Measuring the Impact of Specific Programs

If a state government requires schools to report to parents on their child's body mass index, will it result in lower rates of childhood obesity over time? If frail elders are given an option to hire their adult children or neighbors as caregivers instead of requiring the elders to use formal long-term care workers, will outcomes improve and costs decrease? If a hospital provides readily accessible translation services for non-English-speaking patients, will they become healthier?

These are the types of questions that can be answered through carefully designed program evaluations. For many years, the Foundation has funded independent researchers at universities and other organizations to conduct studies that assess whether the interventions it has funded improve outcomes. It is not coincidental that the Foundation relies on outside evaluators. Having an external, independent team measuring outcomes keeps the process honest. It is too easy for a foundation's program staff and its grantees to become overinvested in a program and reluctant to admit that they have not achieved the desired result. Moreover, when an intervention is successful, the judgment of an independent team increases the credibility of evaluation findings.

Program evaluations also look at implementation issues to learn why outcomes are reached or not and to document how a grantee goes about working on an initiative. Implementation analyses sometimes can help grantees midstream, and most important, they create a roadmap of do's and don'ts that can help in the replication of successful programs.

Program evaluations funded by the Robert Wood Johnson Foundation generally use social science and epidemiological research design concepts. At the heart of this tier of evaluation is comparison: whenever possible, the evaluation team compares outcomes at sites supported by the Foundation with those at similar sites not supported by the Foundation. In the ideal program evaluation, either random assignment or some other mechanism is used to ensure that the comparison sites are as similar as possible to the Foundation-supported sites.

Over the years, the Foundation has learned how difficult it is to mount evaluations in the real world. The perfect evaluation design is generally elusive, baseline data may not be available, and second-best strategies for selecting comparison groups and measuring outcomes are often necessary. Even with the best of intentions, programs tend to evolve over time as priorities change, expected outcomes are revised, or grantees shift their focus. Tensions between program staff and evaluation team members can complicate the evaluation process, and the burden on grantees and program staff members to meet the needs of evaluators is frequently greater than was projected at the start. Often, the findings that emerge are inconclusive or are reported too late to influence decisions about next steps in the Foundation's grantmaking or to inform public opinion.

Thus, the practical difficulties in carrying out rigorous program evaluations are enormous. The evaluation of the Fighting Back program, a nearly $100 million initiative to foster community coalitions to reduce substance abuse in high-risk neighborhoods, provides a classic case study. The program changed course in midstream; the evaluation began after the program was halfway through; the composition of the communities changed; the program office and the evaluation team could not agree on the indicators to be measured; and when the evaluation was finally completed, its findings were strongly disputed.[2]

Whatever the practical difficulties, evaluations do result in learning. Both the Foundation and those outside it use the results of evaluation to develop programs. SUPPORT and Cash & Counseling offer two examples of the practical use of evaluations.

SUPPORT—the Study to Understand Prognoses and Preferences for Outcomes and Risks of Treatments—tested new approaches to providing care for terminally ill hospitalized patients; it involved patients, their families, nurses, and physicians in determining the kind of care that the patients would receive toward the end of their lives. As the demonstration project was being carried out in five hospitals, there was a sense among those involved in it that patients and their families were in fact making better choices, and that their wishes were being respected more. When the research findings were tabulated, however, clear evidence emerged that patients' wishes were not respected and that their care was no different from that of patients who did not receive the special intervention. These findings led to a fundamental rethinking of end-of-life care and paved the way for a decade of Foundation-funded initiatives to reshape the care of terminally ill patients.

The evaluation of the Cash & Counseling program compared the satisfaction levels of people receiving long-term care services from home health care agencies supported by Medicaid to those of another group that was given the option of using family, friends, or community members to deliver the services. The findings of the evaluation demonstrated much higher satisfaction rates among the people given the new option. Timing and reliability of care, treatment of beneficiaries by caregivers, and performance of tasks by caregivers were also substantially better for this group. The evaluation findings provided a basis for recent legislation that expands the Cash & Counseling approach from a three-state demonstration project to an option available in all fifty states.

Evaluations suggesting that no impact was associated with an initiative have led the Foundation to shift priorities. For example, when an evaluation concluded that a fellowship program to improve the understanding and teaching of health care financing was ineffective, the Foundation decided to discontinue the program.[3] Similarly, a negative evaluation of a program to encourage community partnerships to lower the cost of health insurance led the Foundation to end the program and reassess the approach.[4]

The Foundation's long experience in program evaluation has led to numerous lessons, among them:

- It is essential to design programs and evaluations at the same time so that a program can be implemented in a manner that makes an evaluation feasible.

- It is also essential to get timely baseline data if before-and-after comparisons are a feature of an evaluation.

- Evaluation findings need to emerge in a timely manner. Great insights that arrive too late to influence the next steps or federal or state policy have no impact.

- Evaluation design needs to be flexible enough to adjust to changing features of the program being evaluated. Few programs are implemented as planned, and most end up being less ambitious in scope than originally projected.

- The evaluation team and the program team need to work together. Whenever tension, a lack of respect, or an inability to work together characterizes a demonstration initiative, it is unusual for useful findings to emerge.

- Evaluations tend to be stronger when a program has clearly defined and clearly measurable expected outcomes.

—⚬— Tier 2: Performance Indicators: Tracking the Impact of a Portfolio of Programs

Although program evaluations can measure the success or failure of individual programs, the Foundation's trustees and staff want to know what impact its grantmaking in a specific field is having. For example, when the Foundation sets an objective such as reducing tobacco use, they want to know whether smoking has gone down and, to the extent it is possible to know, what contribution the Foundation's programs have made to the decline.

Grantmaking at the Robert Wood Johnson Foundation is mainly directed at attempting to achieve tangible improvement in some aspect of the health system or health-related behavior. The staff and the trustees identify a behavior or public health, health care system, or policy issue that is of concern (such as tobacco use, childhood obesity, or the rising number of uninsured persons), agree upon a specific strategic objective (such as lowering the number of uninsured people by a certain percentage within a specified time period), and then decide on an array of grants that they expect will meet the strategic objective.

To assess whether progress is being made, staff members set down a series of performance indicators that must be reached for the strategic objective to be achieved. These performance indicators are used by the board and the senior staff to judge performance and to guide decisions about resource allocation. Objectives are modified from time to time—often in three- to five-year intervals—but sometimes a priority remains in place for ten or more years.

The performance indicators flow from logic models that the staff develops. These specify, in simple terms, what has to happen in the short and intermediate term if the Foundation can expect to achieve a specified objective in the long run. Short-term indicators are meant to be roughly annual checks on progress that help clarify the Foundation's immediate plans and strategies. A short-term indicator for the tobacco-reduction goal might be convening a summit meeting to help frame policy priorities, followed up by a coordinated plan of action developed by grantees working in this field. Intermediate indicators are measures—often more ambitious than short-term performance indicators—that the Foundation uses to determine progress over a two- to three-year time period. As one example, the Foundation looked at the proportion of the population covered by clean indoor air laws as an intermediate indicator of progress toward its goal of reducing smoking. Long-term indicators reach beyond three years and are broader in focus and level of impact. In the area of tobacco, the Foundation tracked the prevalence of youth smoking as a long-term indicator. Table 5.1 presents a performance indicator report—with short-, medium-, and long-term indicators—that the Foundation staff and board used to track progress in tobacco control.

Each performance indicator—whether short-, intermediate-, or long-term—is also assigned a level of control or influence that indicates how much effect the staff thinks the Foundation can have on reaching it. For example, it is well within the control of the Foundation to organize a meeting of experts on national health insurance, so it would be given a "high" level of control; reducing the number of uninsured by, say, 50 percent depends on factors beyond the Foundation's control and would thus be given a "low" level of control.

Developing this performance assessment system was a major undertaking for the staff. Each internal Foundation team assigned to a specific area of grantmaking was asked to specify the concrete objectives it sought to achieve (such as reducing tobacco use by children, improving retention of nurses, or reducing the disparities among racial or ethnic groups in the care they receive for cardiac conditions). The outcome specified by the objective had to be measurable so that the Foundation's board and the senior staff would know whether the Foundation's grantmaking had had an impact.

The performance measures serve as signposts that help the staff and the board assess whether or not positive change is likely to occur over the long term. If short- and medium-term targets are not met, then the long-term objectives are unlikely to be met as well. The assessment of short- and medium-term objectives can lead the Foundation to alter its strategy (and the logic model guiding it), increase the level of the intervention, or perhaps reconsider the feasibility of reaching the ultimate goal.

Performance measurement is difficult. It is challenging to identify tangible targets that can be measured and that can

Table 5.1.   Strategic Indicators: Tobacco

			Tracking Indicators		
Indicators	**Control**	**Target Date**	**Baseline Status**	**Current Status**	**Target**
State tobacco control funding as a percentage of the CDC minimum (tracking backslide)	M	7/08	40.2% (2000)	22.1% (as of 12/05)	27.0%
Prevalence of cigarette use among 12th graders (tracking backslide)	L	7/08	31.4% (2000)	23.2% (as of 12/05)	25.0%
"Strength of Tobacco Control" Index—monitors tobacco control capacity at state level (tracking backslide)	M	7/08	0 (Normalized/ 2000)	2.4 (as of 12/04)	2.4
Short-term Indicators (4/1/05–4/1/06)	**Control**	**Target Date**	**Baseline Status**	**Current Status**	**Target**
Implemented fund-raising strategy with management	H	7/05	Not completed	Completed (7/05)	To complete
Completed transition plans and budgets for major programs	H	10/05	Not completed	Completed (10/05)	To complete
Intermediate Indicators (13–36 Months)	**Control**	**Target Date**	**Baseline Status**	**Current Status**	**Target**
Combined average state and federal tobacco excise tax	H	7/06	$1.11 (2003)	$1.33 (as of 9/06) Completed (10/05)	$1.25
Proportion of the population covered by comprehensive clean indoor air laws	H	7/06	21.8% (2003)	33.1% (+.09%, 6/06) Partially completed	35.0%
Number of states that cover tobacco dependence treatment through Medicaid (tracking backslide)	L	7/06	38 (2003)	41 (as of 12/05) Completed (12/05)	35

Table 5.1.   Strategic Indicators: Tobacco (*Continued*)

				Tracking Indicators	
Long-term Indicators (+36 Months)	Control	Target Date	Baseline Status	Current Status	Target
Prevalence of youth cigarette use (high school students, grades 9–12)	L	7/07	28.5% (2001)	23.0% (+1.1%, 6/06) Completed (7/04)	23.0%
Prevalence of adult cigarette use	L	7/07	23.2% (2000)	21.1% (+0.2%, early release data as of 6/06)	18.0%
Number of states dedicating CDC-recommended amounts of MSA/tax dollars for tobacco prevention/control	L	7/08	4 (2003)	4 (as of 12/05)	10

Control: L = Low, M = Medium, H = High
Source: Report to the board of trustees of the Robert Wood Johnson Foundation, October 2006.

actually change in the short or intermediate run but do not seem trivial. In managing the process, there is constant concern that focusing on measurable outcomes could lead the Foundation to address less important, though more easily measurable, problems or to adopt less risky program strategies.

The Foundation uses the performance measurement system to force more systematic thinking and to present clear choices. It also forces the staff to concentrate on common, agreed-upon goals. Although the performance measurement system provides guidance for decision making and resource allocation, it is not followed slavishly. The board is sometimes willing to approve grant initiatives even knowing that it will prove difficult to measure the results of the Foundation's investment. For example, it is difficult to demonstrate concrete results of the Foundation's human capital portfolio, but the Foundation's staff and board believe that it is important. Of course, there are critics on both sides of the Foundation's approach to performance measurement. Some at the Foundation feel that the system drives out attention to important objectives that are difficult to quantify. Others feel that the Foundation still does not insist enough on measuring impact in some areas of its grantmaking.

—ᴧᴧ— Tier 3: The Scorecard: Assessing Organizational Effectiveness

The Foundation's annual scorecard has become an integral part of its self-assessment—a tool for senior management, the staff, and the board to assess how the Foundation is doing in a number of areas. It creates a time for formal reflection on the organization's performance and also provides staff members and trustees with a method of identifying and addressing weak areas of organizational performance. For more than a decade, the scorecard has represented an important tool for holding the Foundation accountable to its mission and its guiding principles.

In creating its balanced scorecard, the Foundation adapted a concept developed by the Harvard Business School professor Robert S. Kaplan and the businessman David P. Norton for measuring performance in the business world.[5] Typically, in the business sector these measurements include financial, internal business, innovation and learning, and customers. The Robert Wood Johnson Foundation, whose bottom line is social change rather than profitability, translated these measurements into program impact, program development, customer (that is, grantee) service, and human/financial capital. It also incorporates, as an appendix, a review of grants management performance.

Program Impact

The first section of the scorecard considers whether the Foundation is meeting the goals it set for itself, by presenting the performance indicators for each portfolio and program area. Performance indicators are summarized in terms of the percentage that were completed on time, late, partly completed, or not competed at all. Some commentary on the stability of the indicators is included here, too—whether small or even major changes were made to any indicators in a particular programming area. Although some amount of change to indicators is to be expected in order to maintain the flexibility to adapt to changes in the environment, a complete lack of stability could indicate a lack of sound programming at the beginning.

Also incorporated in the program impact section are data from external audiences: grantees and outside "thought leaders"—a group that includes heads of prominent health organizations, academics, public health officials, Medicaid officials, federal policymakers, state legislators, and the health media. The Foundation's grantees, who have a wide range of expertise, include health researchers, practitioners, advocates, decision makers, and executives. Their judgments about the Foundation's presence, priorities, and effectiveness are an important gauge for the Foundation. Grantees rate the Foundation's impact in a number of ways, including

- Impact on the field, advancement of knowledge in the field, and effect on public policy in grantees' fields
- Objectivity of programming and disseminated materials
- Skill and knowledge of staff
- Influence of programming and communications on health care leaders and policymakers

Thought leaders are asked similar questions, though they are also specifically asked to rate the Foundation's impact on particular programming areas, such as tobacco use, public health, and health insurance coverage. They are also asked to indicate their confidence in, and the usefulness of, information produced by the Foundation.

The grantee and thought leader survey allows the Foundation to compare itself to other foundations. The Center for Effective Philanthropy conducts the grantee survey and directs similar questions to grantees of the Robert Wood Johnson Foundation and other foundations. The Center can then let the Foundation know how it stacks up with other foundations. The thought leader survey asks respondents to rate the Robert Wood Johnson Foundation with a set of its peers, including the Henry J. Kaiser Family Foundation, the W.K. Kellogg Foundation, the Commonwealth Fund, the Pew Charitable Trusts, the California HealthCare Foundation, and the California Endowment. In sum, this section of the scorecard provides the staff and the board with both internal and external indicators and assessments of the Foundation's impact.

Program Development

The scorecard's program development section examines the strength of the Foundation's programming efforts, such as the soundness of its strategies and whether its interests are in line with those of its grantees, thought leaders, and the public. For example, the program development section reviews whether the public perceives health care as a major priority for the government to address, as well as specific health concerns—such as cost, quality, and the uninsured—to get a sense of whether the public's and the Foundation's priorities are aligned. The reasons for including this information in program development are twofold. First, though Robert Wood Johnson is a private foundation, it considers itself to be accountable to the public interest. Second, information about public perceptions of important health topics—childhood obesity, for example—can help guide the Foundation's programming. Moreover, if a topic is of great concern to public health professionals but does not resonate with the public or policymakers, it is an opportunity for the Foundation to inform the public through its communications efforts.

The program development section also incorporates thought leaders' opinions of various health and health care priorities. In 2006, for example, over 90 percent of thought leaders thought that health insurance coverage was a high or very high priority for the nation.

Finally, information from both thought leaders and grantees helps the Foundation understand whether these constituents feel that it is

- Working on issues important to the United States
- Making long-term commitments to important issues
- Supporting and building leadership in health and health care

Customer Service

The survey of grantees, conducted by the Center for Effective Philanthropy, asks how they feel the Foundation is treating them (see box). Indicators from this survey form the basis of the customer service section of the scorecard and include questions such as these:

- Is the Foundation clear about the types of proposals it will fund?
- Is it clear in communicating its goals and objectives?
- Is it fair throughout the application process and responsive throughout the lifetime of a project?
- Are the Foundation's program officers approachable, courteous, and helpful?
- Is the technical assistance provided by or through the Foundation adequate?

The seriousness with which the Foundation takes this information is illustrated by its response to the grantee survey in 2004 that indicated its customer service was not up to that of other foundations. This led to an internal "quality improvement initiative" that resulted in an almost complete overhaul of the Foundation's grant review and approval procedures and the way in which staff members communicated with grantees and potential grantees.

Staff Satisfaction and Financial Performance

This section of the scorecard looks first within the Foundation to determine what the staff thinks of it as a place to work (see box).

This includes information about the staff's overall satisfaction, its ratings of management, and its opinion of its ability to communicate concerns up through the ranks of the Foundation.

This section of the scorecard also reports on how the investment portfolio is doing. The indicators include the return rate and the volatility of the Foundation's endowment portfolio.

The Grantee, Thought Leader, and Public Opinion Surveys

The *grantee survey* asks approximately three hundred grantees about key aspects of the Foundation's service, programs, and impact. It contains questions on

- Grantees' perceptions of the Foundation's impact on their organizations and their field

- Whether the Foundation is addressing the most important health and health care issues and is willing to commit the time and the resources needed to achieve its goals

- How fair the staff is in its interactions with grantees

- Whether the grant application and reporting requirements are burdensome

- How clearly the Foundation communicates its goals and strategies

The survey is confidential and allows for comparisons over time. Recently, it has allowed for comparisons with other funders because of the Foundation's participation in a survey fielded by the Center for Effective Philanthropy that elicits similar information from a number of foundations. Finally, the Foundation periodically surveys applicants it has turned down to look for warning signals coming from this group.

The *thought leader survey* interviews decision makers from universities, health plans, hospitals, health associations, government, the media, and public health organizations. Those in this group are questioned about their knowledge of the Robert Wood Johnson Foundation as an organization and their views on its priorities, its reputation, and the quality of the information it produces. Those who are familiar with the Foundation are asked to rate its impact in addressing problems related to health and health care as well as the impact of its specific strategic areas (for example, quality of care or health insurance coverage). This survey is also confidential, and it, too, allows for comparisons over time.

The *public opinion survey* queries the public about their views on the top issues facing the nation and the Foundation's priorities. Respondents are asked to list the issues they think the government should be addressing and to rate the American health care and public health systems. They are also asked to name the top medical care and public health concerns facing the nation. The survey then asks respondents to rank the Foundation's areas of interest and a few other select health care issues.

The staff survey, which is also confidential, asks staff members how well they think the Foundation is doing in meeting its guiding principles—a core set of values that promote good stewardship of Foundation resources, fairness in the treatment of grantees and the field, and professional, ethical staff conduct. The staff survey asks a number of questions to determine whether staff members feel that the guiding principles are honored by the leadership of the Foundation and are useful in guiding everyday transactions. It also asks questions related to the working environment at the Foundation and the staff's judgment of the Foundation's program development and impact. For example, staff members are asked whether sufficient effort is made to get their opinions, whether there is an environment of teamwork at the Foundation, and whether the Foundation has clear goals and objectives.

Grants Management Performance

The scorecard also contains, as an appendix, a review of data from the Foundation's grants management system to see how many applications are being submitted and, ultimately, being funded; and how the work of the Foundation and its grantees is being disseminated in print and on the Web. It also contains a section that outlines changes that were and will be made.

—∿— Tier 4: Grant Results Reports and The Robert Wood Johnson Foundation Anthology Series

The fourth tier of the Robert Wood Johnson Foundation's evaluative activities, which identifies and shares lessons from the Foundation's grantmaking, takes the form of two publication vehicles: the grant results reports and the annual *Robert Wood Johnson Foundation Anthology*. Both take a broader view of evaluation and attempt to share the understanding gained from the Foundation's investments with as wide an audience as possible.

The grant results reports now total more than two thousand distinct reports that are posted on the Foundation's website. The reports are prepared by a team of consulting writers who are asked to interview key players involved in the grant, read the written record, and prepare a report that summarizes what was actually done with the grant funds and what findings, results, and lessons learned emerged. The reports attempt to tell the stories in a manner that lets the reader come to conclusions about what the facts and experiences suggest about success and failure. The grant results reports unit has recently started to prepare topic summaries, also posted on the Foundation's website, that synthesize the key outcomes and lessons from reports on a particular topic, such as positive youth development or consumer choice in long-term care.

The grant results reports have emerged as the second most visited area of the Foundation's website (just behind the section that describes how to apply for funding). The reports are read by people doing research or planning an initiative that replicates one supported by the Foundation in the past, people interested in knowing what the Foundation funds, and the Foundation's staff members attempting to learn from past lessons to guide current grantmaking.

The Robert Wood Johnson Foundation Anthology, published annually by Jossey-Bass, examines approximately ten topics each year. These topics may be an area of grantmaking, such as health insurance or tobacco policy, or a specific program. Or, in an effort to demystify philanthropy, they may provide an insider's view of how the Foundation reached decisions or chose one path over another. The writers include award-winning journalists, Foundation staff members, and outside evaluators.

The authors sift through the written record, interview key players, and make site visits. They are asked to write an interesting, jargon-free chapter that lets readers know why the Foundation decided to fund the activity, what the program or programs actually did (or are doing, in the case of existing programs), what has been accomplished, and what lessons can be drawn. The book is distributed to more than ten thousand health care experts, foundation staff members and trustees, and government officials, and is available on the Foundation's website.

Taken as a whole, the *Anthology* series, the grant results reports, and publications that emerge from Foundation-funded evaluators (their reports are also available on the Foundation's website) offer an extensive record of the Foundation's successes and failures. Serving as a guide to policymakers, health care leaders, researchers, Foundation staff members, and the general public, they represent one way in which the Foundation tries to be accountable to the public and transparent in its grantmaking.

—ᴡ— An Assessment

The Foundation prides itself on learning from its programs and its evaluations, constantly attempting to improve how it learns. The evolution of the Foundation's evaluation—from evaluation of individual programs to assessments of the impact of portfolios of grants and the production of an internal scorecard—demonstrates the importance of an institutional culture that promotes continual questioning and desire to learn from past experience.

Even so, the practice of evaluation, assessment, and learning still faces challenges. For example, in its traditional program evaluation, the Foundation needs to be sure that the programs it funds to test new ideas are actually designed so that a convincing test can be conducted. A culture such as that of the Robert Wood Johnson Foundation that wants to choose the best grantees and the best programs—rather than comparing a demonstration site with a control site—can actually work against learning. From a strict learning perspective, sites should be chosen so that a legitimate comparison can be made between places that try an idea and places that do "normal practice."

Another challenge is rationing evaluation dollars so they are spent on cases for which testing and learning are possible. Evaluations are often expensive, and confidentiality requirements and the difficulty of collecting survey data have increased their cost in recent years. When a program is not designed to test a new idea, no evaluation may be needed. The decision not to evaluate needs to be made more frequently in order to have money available for more comprehensive evaluations for which testing is possible.

Determining whether a set of Foundation investments have had a causal effect remains a challenge. Currently, performance assessment measures correlation more than causation. Correlation can imply causality when the Foundation's investments are significant enough to be the only likely cause of some event or change. But when the Foundation attempts to affect a complex social situation—such as reducing smoking or improving the quality of health care—it is difficult to know the extent to which the Foundation is responsible for the improvements or whether other factors are the cause.

It is insufficient simply to say that when something positive happens related to a grant program that it is because of the Foundation or its grantees. This expanded sense of impact can be spurious at best. To assess success or failure, the program staff members must be able to articulate the link between the strategy and the expected short-, medium-, and long-term outcomes. Without this type of roadmap, clear assessments will never emerge.

Similarly, the durability of strategy must be considered. On the one hand, it is important for strategy to be flexible enough to react to changes in the environment. On the other hand, if strategies and indicators of success or failure change frequently, then performance assessment is not possible. Constant changes in direction—as opposed to the fine-tuning of a set strategy—generally indicate that a strategy is not working, is not being executed effectively, or was misguided from the start.

Finally, efforts to judge whether the organization itself is working efficiently and effectively require a blend of qualitative assessment and quantitative assessment. The current Robert Wood Johnson Foundation approach perhaps relies too much on quantitative indicators. If the Foundation really wants to know how it is doing, it may need to take the approach of former New York City Mayor Ed Koch and ask in plain language, "How're we doing?" There are many Robert Wood Johnson Foundation–watchers across the country; frank conversations with them could round out the information that the thought leaders' survey provides. Such qualitative information could add an important dimension for the Foundation's board of trustees and senior staff to consider when assessing organizational effectiveness.

The path to developing more effective ways to track and assess performance is the same one the Foundation advises for improving health care quality: continuous quality improvement. Constructing a viable evaluation strategy for a philanthropy is not a one-time building project. It takes constant attention, tinkering, and questioning. While the Robert Wood Johnson Foundation can take pride in its leadership in the field of philanthropic evaluation, it needs to learn from its peers, understand emerging trends in performance assessment, and remain open to evolution in its approaches.

Notes

1. Lavizzo-Mourey, R. "Foreword." *To Improve Health and Health Care: The Robert Wood Johnson Foundation Anthology*, Vol. VII. San Francisco: Jossey-Bass, 2004.
2. Wielawski, I. "Fighting Back." *To Improve Health and Health Care: The Robert Wood Johnson Foundation Anthology*, Vol. VII. San Francisco: Jossey-Bass, 2004.
3. Colby, D. C. "Building Research Capacity in the Sciences." *To Improve Health and Health Care: The Robert Wood Johnson Foundation Anthology*, Vol. VI. San Francisco: Jossey-Bass, 2003.
4. Brown, L. D. and McLaughlin, C. "Constraining Costs at the Community Level: A Critique." *Health Affairs*, 1990, *9*(4), 5–28.
5. Kaplan, R. S. and Norton, D. P. *The Balanced Scorecard: Translating Strategy in Action*. Cambridge, MA: Harvard Business School Press, 1996.

CHAPTER 6

Communications at the Robert Wood Johnson Foundation: Turning Up the Volume, Adjusting the Frequency

Frederick G. Mann and David J. Morse

Editors' Introduction

"Foundations have been slower to integrate communications into their institutional planning and work than any other class of organizations," Frank Karel wrote in the 2001 volume of the *Anthology*.[1] As the Foundation's vice president of communications between 1974 and 1987 and again between 1993 and 2001, Karel almost singlehandedly brought communications into the mainstream of the Foundation's work and helped it realize the vision of communications as an integral part of everything it does. The Foundation's leadership in strategic communications influenced the field to such an extent that many of the country's large foundations now have active communications departments.

Under Karel, the Foundation's communications activities tended to remain in the background, reflecting the preference of both the trustees and the Foundation's presidents—David Rogers, Leighton Cluff, and Steven Schroeder—to "speak through its grantees." As the Foundation gravitated under Risa Lavizzo-Mourey's presidency toward an approach emphasizing social change, its leadership recognized that the Foundation's reputation as a source of trustworthy and unbiased information could play an important role in furthering its policy objectives. As a result, the Foundation's "brand" became more publicly visible, and the Foundation tended to work "with" grantees rather than "through" them. In this reprint, which originally appeared in Volume XIII of the *Anthology*, Fred Mann, the assistant vice president for communications, and David Morse, the vice president for communications from 2001 through mid-2011, describe the use of strategic communications at the Robert Wood Johnson Foundation and trace its evolution over time.

Mann and Morse touch briefly on the use of social media. Although their chapter is only three years old, since the time it was published, the Foundation has undergone a revolution as it has taken advantage of advances in communications technology and become a "Web 2.0 foundation." In addition to the many tools that Mann and Morse highlight in their chapter, the Foundation is now communicating with new audiences through social media, such as Facebook, Twitter, and blogs, and through its website, www.rwjf.org.

Note

1. Karel, F. "Getting the Word Out: A Foundation Memoir and Personal Journey." *To Improve Health and Health Care 2001: The Robert Wood Johnson Foundation Anthology*. San Francisco, Jossey-Bass, 2001.

I t's not easy to build on the work of a master. Oh, sure, a lot of the heavy lifting has been done for you, and many of the pivotal early battles have been won. But trying to follow in the large footsteps of a well-known leader in any field is a difficult mission at best.

In our case, the field is foundation communications, and the leader whose vision we are attempting to keep current and adapt to changing times is Frank Karel, longtime vice president for communications at the Robert Wood Johnson Foundation and at the Rockefeller Foundation, former program officer at the Commonwealth Fund, former journalist, and, in the eyes of many, the man who almost single-handedly raised the stature and the strategic importance of communications throughout the foundation world.

Back in 2001, just before he retired (for the second time) from the Robert Wood Johnson Foundation, Karel wrote for this *Anthology* series about how our foundation's communications efforts had evolved over the years.[1] "Foundations have been slower to integrate communications into their institutional planning and work than any other class of organizations in our society," he wrote. Commenting on the congressional hearings leading up to passage of the Tax Reform Act of 1969—sweeping legislation that affected the operation of private foundations, many of which had taken a public beating, he noted: "The prevailing mood and mindset in the foundation world was to keep as quiet and as low a public profile as possible."

Karel set out to change that mindset. He brought a modern sense of communications to this foundation and others, and he helped put strategic communications planning and practice in the center ring of philanthropic work. "Communications has become an integral part of everything we do," he wrote in his 2001 *Anthology* chapter. "The aim is to share our vision of using communications strategically—that is to create and use information in ways that can help achieve key organizational and program objectives."

We have tried to build on Karel's firm footing and, as he did, align communications efforts with the Foundation's objectives. But as those objectives and strategies have evolved over the years, so, too, has our approach to communications. Today our programs focus largely on influencing and changing public policy and organizational practice to improve the health and health care of all Americans. The key tools we use for influence are advocacy, public education, and communications. We advocate for change. We inform policy debates. We have more targeted and time-delineated goals focused on bringing about positive improvements in people's lives. Our big-issue approach to improve health care quality, to reverse the childhood obesity epidemic, to build and fortify public health systems, and to provide affordable and stable health insurance coverage for all has made influencing public policies and systems vital to us.

"It is through policy change that societies make and remake themselves," the Foundation's senior vice president for health, James Marks, and the journalist Joseph Alper wrote in their chapter "Shaping Public Policy as a Robert Wood Johnson Foundation Approach" in Volume XII of this series. "With limited philanthropic resources available, working to change policy offers foundations the possibility of improving the lives of many more people than they could through other forms of grantmaking, such as direct services grants. And the improvements are likely to be longer lasting since once enacted, policy remains and becomes part of the societal landscape. For foundations, this represents social change and one of the most effective ways they can leverage their investments."[2]

Today the Foundation has a voice in the policy arena. And we want that voice to be heard. Our megaphone is our new communications model—a direct descendant of Frank Karel's "getting the word out" approach, but now a more strategic, centralized, policy reform-focused system that does more than just complement our programmatic objectives; it is essential to actually bringing about the lasting social change we seek.

Of course, as Frank Karel noted, cranking up the communications volume and effectiveness does not come naturally in the foundation world. Foundations can be quiet places. Ours certainly often seems to be.

Foundation staff members don't sell products or maximize revenue. Instead, their fundamental purpose is to make a difference in people's lives. As far as work with a purpose goes, this is the top of the scale. You'd think the people who got to do this would be singing and dancing and throwing confetti on the way out of the door each night. But that's not the foundation culture. People at most foundations do love their work and know that the impact they have to improve the lives of others can be huge. But the workplace is usually dignified, polite, and scholarly, not showy or boisterous. When Rebecca Rimel, the president and CEO of The Pew Charitable Trusts, was once asked by a visitor why her foundation was so quiet, she replied, "Yes, we're a bit like ducks you see gliding quietly and effortlessly across a pond, but if you look just below the surface, you see those webbed feet paddling furiously. So it's quiet at the surface, but not so quiet below."

Still, it seems pretty quiet in areas where communications officers congregate. Their counterparts in print, broadcast, and online newsrooms may celebrate a great series with high fives and war whoops (and a truly notable achievement like a Pulitzer Prize with sprayed champagne), but foundations and their communications staffs are far more circumspect. As Joel Fleishman noted in his insightful 2007 book *The Foundation: A Great American Secret*, "Foundations have generally shared a 'culture of diffidence' that discourages openness about their activities and agendas."[3] This diffidence, he writes, stems in part "from a long-prevalent sense that it is unseemly for a charitable giver to 'toot his own horn' by publicizing his gifts. For many tradition-minded philanthropoids, even issuing press releases about their grants feels uncomfortably like bragging."

So imagine the odd scene the morning of April 4, 2007, when the staff of the Robert Wood Johnson Foundation gathered around a large projected image of their president and CEO Risa Lavizzo-Mourey—and cheered her appearance on NBC's *Today* show. She was there to promote the Foundation's very public announcement that it would devote $500 million over the next five years to reverse the nation's dangerous childhood obesity epidemic.

The announcement went far beyond the comfy couches of *Today*. As envisioned in a plan drawn up by Adam Coyne, the Foundation's director of public affairs, *The New York Times* carried a lengthy exclusive story about the Robert Wood Johnson Foundation's ambitious childhood obesity pledge; the Associated Press wrote a story that ran in scores of papers around the country; Lavizzo-Mourey and other Foundation representatives appeared on the nightly network news shows, PBS's *NewsHour with Jim Lehrer*, NPR (National Public Radio), and other key news outlets.[4] The Foundation laid the groundwork by sending information on the Foundation's commitment to more than 800 reporters covering health, health care, and philanthropy; distributing a video package to more than 200 television and radio stations nationwide; updating the Foundation website; posting an electronic letter to more than 25,000 grantees and website content subscribers; and contacting every member of Congress, every governor and lieutenant governor, mayors in the 100 largest cities, members of state legislatures' health committees, and federal agencies and organizations.

—∿— The Way We Were and Why We've Changed

Given Frank Karel's strong guidance, the Robert Wood Johnson Foundation was never particularly shy when it came to communicating. Under Karel's leadership, the Foundation's communication department grew in both size and mission. Communications became integral to Foundation programs, and communications staff people were full members of Foundation program teams. Communications-related grants, largely for the Campaign for Tobacco-Free Kids to reduce smoking among teens and for ads produced for the Partnership for a Drug-Free America, grew significantly, and accounted for more than 20 percent of all funds awarded by the Foundation from 1997 to 2001.

But even as communications took a central role within the Foundation, the messages reaching the outside world could be somewhat scattered, and sometimes even contradictory. For most of the Foundation's history, our explicit approach to communicating about mission, goals, strategies, and objectives had been that "we speak through our grantees." That approach was expressed a decade ago by then-president Steven Schroeder in a statement of core values and commitments. But even as he affirmed this grantee-centered communications strategy, Schroeder noted drawbacks to the approach—that speaking indirectly through many grantees who themselves have different objectives made it more difficult for the Foundation to "influence the policy process" and that "we pay a price in the potential attenuation of policy leverage."

Our influence in shaping change in health and health care, therefore, has been derivative historically, since our grantees were our principal agents who executed Robert Wood Johnson Foundation strategies. Having multiple voices delivering multiple messages on different issues (or even the same issue) was harder for key audiences to process than sending consistent messages from consistent sources. Furthermore, when the Robert Wood Johnson Foundation spoke about an issue—like health insurance coverage, tobacco, or end-of-life care—primarily through grantees, it was difficult for those receiving messages to know the overarching goals and objectives of the Foundation, the nature of its role and relationship to a grantee, and the salience of the issue to the Foundation, policymakers, and the public.

Grantee-centered communications made perfect sense when the Foundation was initiating and funding national programs and projects that were loosely related to one another within broadly defined fields: access; quality; addiction prevention; and healthy communities and lifestyles—its goal areas in the 1990s and early 2000s. But today our programming is more targeted, rewording for awk driving us toward measurable social change in policy, in organizational practice, and in behavior. In 2003, Risa Lavizzo-Mourey assumed the presidency of the Foundation and developed an "Impact Framework," which continues to guide our programs to this day. This framework organized the Foundation's philanthropic investments through a set of diversified portfolios, much like those of mutual funds, to meet short-term, medium-term, and long-term goals. This structure has brought a sharp focus to how we try to solve pressing health and health care problems, and has also given us the means to more effectively manage and measure the results of our work.

The Impact Framework also required a different approach to communications—one that emphasizes the Foundation's speaking collaboratively *with* our grantees and other colleagues in addressing the issues that are the pillars of the framework—like the need for health coverage for all Americans and rolling back the tide of childhood obesity. Rather than embedding communications resources directly in each major grant, with each grantee communicating independently, we have shifted our communications approach to intentionally speaking together and collaboratively *with* our grantees rather than *through* them—viewing grantees and the Foundation as an interdependent family of people and programs with common goals and common messages.

Communications dollars that used to be included in grants so that grantees could independently promote their work and publicize their findings and their accomplishments are now largely held back and are spent at the Foundation level. Instead of grantees issuing statements and releasing white papers that could step on the toes of other grantees working in the same field, messaging and timing of communications is now coordinated centrally by the Robert Wood Johnson communications staff. The result is greater efficiency and, we believe, greater impact.

As we took these steps—centralizing communications strategy and messaging, speaking collaboratively with grantees, tying communications objectives closely to our philanthropic program goals—we were doing something new and unlikely for us: putting ourselves in the spotlight along with our grantees. Not because we sought more ink but, rather, because we sought a paradigm shift in the conventional wisdom about philanthropy generally and the Robert Wood Johnson Foundation's philanthropy specifically: to accelerate and accentuate a shift in perception from simply being a *grantmaker*, or provider of funds for good works, to that of a catalyst, expert, and leader in creating systemic change and improvement in health and health care.

In a 1998 *Health Affairs* article, Steven Schroeder not only restated his "we speak through our grantees" philosophy but also added, "(we) do not seek a high institutional profile. We have chosen to work primarily through our grantees, rather than establish ourselves as a primary source of information." A decade later, we and our grantees firmly believe that we can have a greater collective impact if the Foundation speaks and stands *with* them rather than speaking *through* them.[5]

The strategy for maximizing our communications impact is fairly simple. First, create common, closely aligned communications on behalf of issues that we, grantees, and colleagues are addressing together—like rolling back childhood obesity, creating greater quality and equality in health care, and improving the health of vulnerable people by attacking the social factors that impede their health. Second, link these communications across programs and issues into a more comprehensive approach, one that we hope is a more robustly influential Robert Wood Johnson Foundation in which the whole is more than the sum of the parts.

Enhancing our influence as a health and health care leader and leveraging our impact fully requires us to speak more authoritatively as a foundation, to strengthen our credibility as a source of essential information about changing policy and practice, to attract significant and influential partners, to add value to our grantees' work and reputation, and to elevate our stature as a guiding force and catalyst for change in health and health care.

—⚯— It Began with a Promise

Discovering the benefit of building our own image and speaking directly for causes we champion was not a quick or easy process. It started with the idea of identifying the Foundation's brand—what the Foundation was and why we were in the business we were in. As long ago as 2002, President Schroeder brought together twenty-five staff members from all levels of the organization, along with a few members of the Foundation's board of trustees, to ascertain the characteristics of our Foundation's brand. To even consider that a philanthropy had a brand was unprecedented: brands were seen as the province of the corporate world, and of large nonprofit organizations that provided direct benefits, like education, health care, and social services. We had a mission statement, well-articulated goals, and a tag line (most often heard on NPR), but we didn't have, or didn't think we had, a brand.

At Schroeder's five-hour evening meeting, people sat at a large, open-square table, each with a laptop computer, for what Dave Richardson, president of Wirthlin Worldwide (now Harris Interactive), the lead facilitator of the session, called an Advanced Strategy Lab. Richardson started by describing what a brand and branding were: "management of actions and communications with constituents to move them from what they *currently* think of your organization to how *you want them* to think of the organization." In other words, according to Richardson, branding is about being known for attributes *we* (the organization) would like *you* (our audience or constituents) to know about. He then peppered the group with questions. Each person entered brief answers on a laptop, and then viewed their collective responses almost immediately on a large screen at the front of the room. His first question was simple: "What business are you in?" The dominant answer was simple, too: "We're in the grantmaking business." Richardson paused and asked the question again: "What business are you in?" Again the same answer. But he clearly expected a different response, so he asked a slightly different question: "Is grantmaking the *purpose* of your business or is it *what* you do?"

You could almost see the collective light bulbs going on over the heads around the room, and could see them literally on the screen at the front: "Aha, we're in the social change business—the business of improving health and health care for all Americans. Grantmaking is what we do—a means to our goals, not why we do it."

It was clear that the group, all insiders, considered the Robert Wood Johnson Foundation to be essentially a bank or a philanthropic ATM machine—you put your card in, in the form of a grant application and, after some due diligence, you got your money (or not, if your application was turned down). And that was conventional wisdom about foundations, from both inside and outside the philanthropic world—that we were essentially *transactional* organizations.

That was certainly the way the public—through the prism of the press—saw us. A recent survey by InfoTrend of 40,000 news stories mentioning foundations since 1990 showed that 99 percent of those stories were about transactions—grants made or paid—and not about foundations' or even their grantees' impact.[6]

Recognizing that the transactional brand we thought we had wasn't the one we wanted to have was hard. In 2002 and 2003, we organized similar branding labs with grantees, representatives of media organizations, and policy leaders. Ironically, they understood that the Foundation's mission was about catalyzing social change in health and health care better than the Foundation staff who participated in that first lab. They recognized that our greatest asset was our reputation for objective data, building evidence, and creating influence for change, not simply the dollars we provided.

And then we conducted the labs with the entire staff, and finally developed a set of characteristics that reflected, we think, both what the Foundation was and what we aspired to be. It reflected more about what others thought of us and what we should be than what we had thought of ourselves. But we still couldn't call it our brand, since that would be too "commercial," according to most of the staff. We called it the Robert Wood Johnson Foundation Promise.

The Robert Wood Johnson Foundation Promise

We care deeply about the pressing health and health care issues that this country faces. When issues of national magnitude—like covering the uninsured, improving the care of chronic illnesses, developing the next generation of leaders, improving the health of the most vulnerable among us, revamping our public health system—need leadership, the Robert Wood Johnson Foundation has traditionally stepped forward.

The reason isn't simply that significant issues need significant resources. For thirty-five years, we've brought not just our financial assets, but our deep experience, commitment and a rigorous, balanced approach to the problems that affect both the health care and the health of all those we serve.

We focus on issues that demand attention. We work with a diverse group of people whose dedication, expertise and perspective lead to sound, new solutions. We will not shy away from difficult or controversial questions. And we have the staying power to stick with problems until solutions become clear, momentum has been established, and progress has been made.

We believe in supporting programs that have measurable impact and that create meaningful and timely change—helping Americans lead healthier lives and get the care they need—because we expect to make a difference in your lifetime.

Moving from a principal mindset of being basically a grant-maker to seeking impact and influence in health and health care hasn't been without challenges, and it hasn't happened overnight.

It took two years before we could even consider moving from using the "Promise" euphemism (although it's not a bad one) to using the "B" word. But there is increasing comfort, among both staff and grantees, with the concept of a Foundation brand and, more importantly, with its implementation. Results in 2008 from our annual "Scorecard" survey of health experts, business leaders, and policymakers suggest that these key

Foundation constituencies resonate with core characteristics of the Robert Wood Johnson Promise. They believe that the Foundation addresses important, difficult issues in health and health care; that we stick with addressing long-standing problems; and that we're objective and rigorous.[7]

—∽— A Culture of Storytelling

We think, as did Frank Karel, that the best way of getting the word out about the Foundation, our grantees, and our collective impact is by telling stories about our work and about the people we are trying to serve. As our colleague Andy Goodman describes in *Storytelling as Best Practice*, while evidence—the "cold hard facts"—is critical to making one's case, it's the story, supported by evidence, that convinces and moves one to action. In his introduction to Goodman's monograph, Ira Glass, the founder and host of public radio's *This American Life*, a mecca for storytelling, notes, "The most powerful thing you can hear, and the only thing that ever persuades any of us in our own lives, is [when] you meet somebody whose story contradicts the thing you think you know. At that point, it's possible to question what you know, because the authenticity of their experiences is real enough to do it." Richard Wirthlin, the communications guru and adviser to Ronald Reagan, a consummate storyteller, put it more simply: that people are persuaded rationally but motivated emotionally.

Goodman, a Foundation grantee, thinks so: "To evaluate how well an organization communicates, I start by looking at how well it tells stories about its work. I don't care how big they are or how many resources they have at their disposal—if they can't tell a good story, then they haven't mastered the most fundamental form of human communication." He notes that the Robert Wood Johnson Foundation is developing a culture of storytelling, and, even better, insisting that its grantees do so as well. "Now, this doesn't mean that Robert Wood Johnson doesn't rely on data to make its case; like most foundations, it is awash in numbers," he says. "But its program officers and staff use stories as the spear point to pierce the veil of apathy (or distraction, or the numbness of information saturation) and get their audience's full attention. And once they have that attention, then they present the data to show there is more than one story to be told."

—∿— Measuring Up

"The Robert Wood Johnson Foundation today understands that communications means more than just publishing a report. It is really about creating a simple, compelling message that can get people to change their behavior," says Bruce Siegel, a physician who is the director of the Center for Health Care Quality at the Department of Health Policy at George Washington University School of Public Health and Health Services. "Sometimes this means targeting patients, other times nurses or CEOs. But it is still about helping someone to understand that they need to do things differently."

Siegel, a former New Jersey commissioner of health, who has served as the director of several Robert Wood Johnson Foundation national programs, says that the Foundation's staff members "work hand in glove with their expert partners to understand a problem as well as its solutions. Then they seek to use the entire array of media to spread a consistent message that can move people to action. A big part of this process is absolute honesty: the goal here is to figure out what really works, not just what makes us feel good about ourselves."

But how do we know what really works? How will we know if we have really done our job well? How do we measure progress toward our goals? In certain instances, measuring the success of a communications effort is pretty easy. Take the childhood obesity announcement. We had newspaper clips to read and television news tapes to watch. We saw traffic on the Foundation's website spike to new levels, and we had phones ringing off the wall with calls from people eager to help us spend the $500 million we had pledged. But without clear and precise strategic programming and communications plans to spend that huge sum of money wisely and effectively, a raised Foundation profile is just an easy target at which critics will shoot.

Our program team working on reversing the childhood obesity epidemic by the year 2015 has those strategic plans—and more. For example, it is actively pushing for policy changes on the national, state, and local levels that will improve the nutritional quality of food served in schools, reinstate physical education, and improve the access to affordable fresh food and safe places for children to play in poor and vulnerable communities. They are funding studies, convening experts, and creating a new hub of knowledge and action for the field in the Robert Wood Johnson Foundation Center to Prevent Childhood Obesity. With the new center, they are helping to create an online community that will serve as the go-to resource for our major community-based action and advocacy programs, *Healthy Kids, Healthy Communities*, and *Communities Creating Healthy Environments*, as well as our other grantees and the obesity-prevention field at large. There is substance backing up the $500 million public pledge.

"The legitimacy and persuasiveness of a foundation's voice in its efforts to influence public policy depends entirely on the evidence-based knowledge and carefully-researched program demonstrations with which it can buttress its views," says Joel Fleishman, author of *The Foundation* and professor of Law and Public Policy at Duke University. "Unless backed up by evidence that persuades, a foundation's voice is just another person's opinion. What infuses the Robert Wood Johnson Foundation's communications efforts with great credibility are the thirty-eight years of consistent devotion to finding out and documenting the extent to which its grantmaking initiatives have indeed been effective, and to sharing its findings with the professional community and the public. That honesty and that openness are what give great weight and influence to the Robert Wood Johnson Foundation's efforts to persuade the public, the policymakers and the relevant professions."

Not all communications efforts, however, are as clear to measure—or so certain to have impact or be noticed as having impact—as pledging to give away $500 million.

If you're in the business of being a philanthropic bank, measurement of success seems fairly simple: numbers of grants made, dollars out the door to meet annual required payout, geographic and demographic distribution of grant funds—all can be counted. But if you're in the business of measuring social change, outcome seems far more complex. What's the marginal contribution of a foundation, a grantee, or any other single organization to driving down smoking rates among America's youth, increasing enrollment of eligible kids in the State Children's Health Insurance Program, rolling back the national epidemic of childhood obesity, or improving the quality and equality of health care in, say, Cleveland or Memphis? And can we measure the contribution and the cost-effectiveness of our communications efforts toward those goals? Since we're a health foundation, we often think in the language of prevention and treatment—what's the right formulary and dose of communications to reach a particular goal?

One of our goals over the years has been to ensure that all Americans have affordable, stable health care coverage. There are more than 46 million uninsured people in the United States. With our Foundation's assets, we could probably buy an inexpensive, high-deductible health insurance policy for a few million uninsured Americans for a year. That's easily measurable—but we wouldn't have a foundation anymore. So we've focused on increasing the salience and the political and economic unacceptability of having 46 million uninsured in America. For several years, we have mounted a series of Cover the Uninsured campaigns, with partners like the American Hospital Association, the AFL-CIO, the United States Chamber of Commerce, America's Health Insurance Plans, and others[8] —all organizations that recognize that we can't sustain a society in which tens of millions have no access to high-quality affordable care, but all of which have very different perspectives on how to address the problem of uninsurance.

The campaigns are intended to help change the frame—the perceptive boundary—in which the public, opinion leaders, and policymakers know and understand who the uninsured are. Understanding who they really are, we believe, can increase the propensity of policymakers to act on their behalf. We've done market research, conducted polls and focus groups, tested and retested messages, done pre- and post-campaign analyses. Since these campaigns began, the dominant frame has changed. The research tells us that the public no longer sees the uninsured as simply the downtrodden looking for a handout, but, rather, as people like *you*—parents and kids in working families, your close relatives, your neighbors and friends—who aren't uninsured by choice but because they or their employer can't afford insurance. Americans now know that 80 percent of the uninsured are in working families.

Is that a communications success? While the fundamental goal of stable, affordable coverage for all Americans is still elusive, we seem to have achieved what we believe to be one of the building blocks toward reaching that goal. But what's our foundation's marginal contribution toward creating a new conventional wisdom about the uninsured? We've asked an outside evaluator—a political scientist at the University of Minnesota—to help us answer that question. He will report back to us in a few months.

Some communications professionals say it's okay to measure "contribution rather than attribution." A former boss calls it "plausible connectivity"—a reasonable link between what we sought to do and the desired outcome, even if there's a lot of noise in the system that makes it difficult, if not impossible, to tease out the marginal contribution. Perhaps. But we are still searching for that magic measurement bullet.

By one measurement, it appears as if our new communications approach is reaping benefits. According to a content analysis of articles in the top twenty-five American newspapers, long-lead magazines (like *Time* and *Newsweek*), and health trade journals, of 1,400 articles reviewed between 2003 and 2008 that mention the

Foundation, 26 percent (370) associated the Robert Wood Johnson Foundation with specific brand attributes—our leadership, strategies, partnerships with key players, policy aims and outcomes—rather than simply transactions. (It's a nice improvement over the InfoTrend study showing 99 percent of stories about all foundations being strictly about transactions.) This analysis, conducted by CARMA International, states that the brand attributes most associated with the Foundation were leadership, making a positive difference in people's lives, successful partnerships, policy influence, and taking a strategic approach to meeting its mission. These data reflect media coverage in only a few specific, albeit important, print media—not broadcast, cable, Web, and other electronic and social media that we know are increasingly where the general public and opinion leaders connect and get their information. But we view the print content analysis as a positive sign not just that our Foundation messaging is being heard but also that we seem to be growing our impact and influence.

—⁓— Growing Electronically

Our main vehicle for sharing information about impact is our website and the electronic media strategy that undergirds it. Like many other foundations, we are aligning our communications model to take advantage of the new interactive features and functionalities that social media and Web 2.0 technologies provide. Foundations have never been early adopters, but they have been using websites to promote their grantees and their work for many years. Now, with the growth of social media, those sites have the capacity to be much more than promotional vehicles and online storage rooms for white papers and grantee reports. Today's technology is all about interactivity. The website is not just the Foundation's front door to the world; it is the home for debate, dialogue, creation, and connection for both the foundation and its audiences. And, happily, it is one form of communications outreach where participation (if not clear success) is measurable.

It's fair to say that back before we changed our communications model and started to see how a website could really build a connection with key audiences and give us a larger voice, our site wasn't as good as it should have been. RWJF.org was hard to navigate, and users found it hard to search for information they wanted and knew was there. There was no clear indication of our priorities; the audiences we particularly wanted to reach—policymakers, opinion leaders, the media, as well as our current and prospective grantees—would have a hard time figuring out what we, the Foundation, thought was most important. Our program teams were more focused on making and managing grants than on collecting and promoting the learning and knowledge gleaned from their work. The website was considered the exclusive province of the Foundation's Communications and Research and Evaluation units.

Since the change to the team-oriented Impact Framework approach and the embracing of the Robert Wood Johnson Foundation brand, program staff members now understand that their role extends beyond just grantmaking. They have increasingly turned to using the website and related electronic media to drive toward meeting team objectives and promoting the learning derived from our philanthropic investments. But despite this important internal conversion—and some good trends that showed a steady growth of our online audience—we were still not doing enough with the Web. One of our program teams, the one working to improve both the quality and equality of health care, was eager to embrace the Web in order to build interest in its issues, share results, and interact with all sides of the health care quality debate. But given the technical and design constraints of RWJF.org, the team could not see the website filling its new needs.

So at the end of 2007 we embarked on a quick but thorough redesign of the Foundation's website to enhance our impact, promote social change, and showcase the knowledge and experience that are core elements of the Foundation's brand. We also did it to take advantage of all of the benefits that the expanding interactive

Web offers. In June 2008, in conjunction with the announcement of the Foundation's $300 million investment to improve quality in health care markets in specific regions across the country, and guided by a new cross-Foundation Editorial Policy Board that sets Web strategy and oversees the quality and focus of our electronic communications products, we relaunched RWJF.org. Its target audiences remained policymakers, policy influencers, state officials, congressional staff, grant seekers, grantees, and the media. And what they found was a site that was more flexible—more able to spotlight goals and developments like the regional health care quality effort—and fresher and newsier, with content changing more frequently to drive repeat user traffic.

We improved the design of the website to better display both the programmatic work of our teams and, in keeping with our new higher profile approach, to show the Foundation's commitment to social change. We improved the site's search and navigation functions so that our large volume of reports, analyses, and evaluations could be more easily found by our Web audience. On the new RWJF.org, visitors can more quickly and easily learn what the Foundation is about and what we deem important. They can continue to receive weekly "news digests" about issues and events in childhood obesity, nursing, health insurance coverage, and other key fields, as well as timely "content alerts" highlighting new developments in research and policy related to public health, vulnerable populations, and quality and equality of care.

In early 2009, with health reform becoming a major issue of interest in Washington, we launched a new Health Reform section of our website. The section continues to grow and serves as a home for comprehensive, balanced, timely information on important reform issues with content being provided not only by Robert Wood Johnson but also by other responsible news sources and by active participants on our health reform blog.

Information across the site is now presented in forms that are easier for Google and other search engines to find and display. Our new internal analytics capacity helps us follow site usage patterns in detail. We can determine who is coming to RWJF.org, where they are coming from, how long they are staying, which reports and publications they are downloading, which program areas and subfields have the most loyal following, and how many visitors are signing up for our news digests and other electronic products.

Knowing how many policymakers and other information seekers are coming to us and what they are interested in is an important measure of the effectiveness of our communications outreach and our programming work. Our editorial policy board and Web team are tracking various metrics carefully to learn what types of content are most valued by our different audiences.

The new website also provides the social media functionality we knew we needed, which allows for greater information sharing and collaboration with grantees and users. We are currently hosting blogs, discussion boards, and interactive chats. We have established a Robert Wood Johnson Foundation presence on YouTube, Twitter, and soon Facebook—the most ubiquitous Web-based social-networking channels. We have syndication (RSS—Really Simple Syndication) feeds available on hundreds of topics and publication types so people can get automatic feeds delivered to them on topics of their choice. And we are integrating these feeds into grantee websites. We are crawling their sites for content we want to display on the Foundation's site, and we are exporting our content to our grantees' sites via "widgets" (pre-branded headline components that allow the Foundation to offer news digests, the latest research and publications, news releases, and other content, sorted by topic). We have also built a "Slidebuilder" in order to easily present charts and PowerPoint presentations from grantees; congressional, state, and local policymakers now are able to download or print them easily and include this Foundation content in their presentations and reports. This has answered a clear need, particularly for our policymaker audience and for others who wanted quick, digestible, graphical information.

We have created a central grantee product repository that allows us to collect publications from our grantees and display them both internally for our staff and externally on RWJF.org. In short, we are building a content distribution network that will turn the Foundation and our major grantee sites into one family with all our knowledge products given maximum distribution, all on behalf of the specific social changes in health and health care we and our grantees and philanthropic colleagues seek—rolling back childhood obesity, securing health care coverage for all Americans, transforming our outmoded public health systems, and improving the quality and equality of care. It's less about tooting our own horn and more about influencing these transformative goals.

—⚬— Connecting with Policymakers

One indication that policymakers are starting to take more notice of your stature in the field is how often they ask not for your money but for your advice. The Robert Wood Johnson Foundation is unique among American foundations in having a formal program to link the Foundation and our grantees directly and strategically with policymakers in Washington and increasingly in the states. It's called the Connect project, and through it the Foundation's leadership and our grantees have become sources of congressional testimony and expert advisers on health and health care matters.

Connect was founded back in 1998 by the ever-forward-thinking Frank Karel and one of his communications officers, Joe Marx. It was designed to help our grantees establish and build relationships with their congressional delegations. Of course, the Foundation is prohibited from lobbying, and our grantees are prohibited from using our funds to lobby. But Connect is not about lobbying—it's about educating members of Congress and their staff about the critical health challenges and creative solutions being developed, tested, and implemented in their states and districts. It's about engaging policymakers to learn about and support these promising projects in non-legislative ways: through site visits, with letters of support, and by connecting grantees to key partners in the community.

Since its inception, Connect has scheduled meetings between hundreds of Robert Wood Johnson grantees and their members of Congress, and has organized dozens of Capitol Hill briefings for congressional staff members to highlight the work of our grantees. Over time, the program has also incorporated a robust training element to ensure that grantees are well prepared with a clear message, a compelling story, and a specific, non-legislative "ask" in each of their meetings, and has provided technical assistance to grantees to ensure that they follow up on those asks effectively when they go back home.

Although a Robert Wood Johnson representative typically accompanies the grantees on their meetings with members of Congress and their staff, and usually leaves behind a list of Foundation-supported projects in the member's state or district, Connect has been solely focused on positioning the grantees—and not the Foundation itself—as resources on the Hill.

As the Foundation shifted its communications approach to speaking *with* our grantees, the Connect project expanded its focus. Although we continue to support our grantees through training, meetings, and briefings on Capitol Hill, we also began, in 2006, to have a more explicit focus on positioning the Foundation itself as a resource to federal policymakers and their staff. Several times each year, senior staff, including our president and CEO (and, occasionally, our board chair) meet with members of Congress both to share our lessons learned and to seek advice from the leaders in Congress on health and health care. These meetings allow us to put the work of our grantees in a broader context and to make connections across the Foundation's program areas.

Reaching out to members of Congress and developing relationships with them and their staff has led to additional opportunities for Robert Wood Johnson Foundation staff members to testify at congressional hearings, in some cases alongside our grantees. For example, in October 2007, Risa Lavizzo-Mourey testified at a House Energy and Commerce Health Subcommittee hearing on tobacco; a Foundation grantee, William Corr, then executive director of the Campaign for Tobacco-Free Kids, was also a witness. In 2007 and 2008, Foundation staff members testified at congressional hearings on childhood obesity, quality, and disparities in health care. Working with the Connect project, Foundation grantees have also testified at hearings on long-term care, school nutrition, and childhood obesity.

Not all of our Connect work is done in Washington. For instance, in 2008, after Foundation communications and program officers provided information to a *Wall Street Journal* reporter about one of our projects—Green House, an innovative alternative to a traditional nursing facility—and a glowing page one article was published, Connect organized a site visit for congressional staff members to a Green House facility. A bipartisan group of House and Senate staff members, as well as staff members from the Congressional Research Service and the Centers for Medicare and Medicaid Services visited the Lebanon Valley Brethren Home in Palmyra, Pennsylvania. There they toured the traditional nursing home on campus, as well as one of the four Green House homes on site to see firsthand the difference in the two settings, and to hear from the home's residents and staff, as well as the national program staff of the Green House initiative. Green Houses, they were told, provide an environment in which residents receive nursing support and clinical care without the care becoming the focus of their existence. By altering the facility size, interior design, staffing patterns, and methods of delivering services to residents, the Green House model provides residents with greater health and lifestyle benefits than do traditional nursing and assisted-living buildings. Early results show that Green House residents report higher satisfaction levels, less physical decline, and less depression.

The visitors heard from Robert Wood Johnson staff members about the Foundation's support for the Green House, and also about our broader commitment to improving long-term care and community-based services for the nation's aging population. Through visits such as this, people making public policy get the opportunity to see the work of Robert Wood Johnson and its grantees and come to understand the role the Foundation can play in helping Americans lead healthier lives and get the care they need.

—⚹— Plans for the Future

Expanding Connect is but one way we hope to keep moving forward with communications efforts aimed at fostering policy change. Through greater content sharing with grantees on the Web and co-branding of grantee and Foundation products electronically and in print, we seek to broaden the distribution of our knowledge and spread awareness about how we can influence policy debates. Our goal is to continually make our communications collaborative, not derivative. Among our specific goals for the next few years are these:

Expand Our Outreach to News Organizations

Establishing a voice for the Foundation is one thing. Having that voice heard is quite another. Robert Wood Johnson was an early foundation supporter of NPR, starting back in 1985, and has continued its support for health reporting from 1986 through the present day. In addition, the Foundation has, since 2005, funded health reporting on PBS' *The NewsHour with Jim Lehrer*, which has been ranked first among all television news programs as the most credible, objective, and influential. The survey further notes that *The NewsHour* is among the leading programs in reaching elite policymakers who directly affect a broad range of health issues.[9] By supporting strong journalism that increases the scope, the quality, and the depth of health and health care reporting, important policy issues are most effectively raised to a more engaged public and to policymakers. For the past ten years, we have also been a major supporter of the Association of Health Care Journalists, feeling that members of this organization are also well positioned to provide accurate, timely news and analysis on issues of importance to the Foundation and its target audiences. These connections help raise the Foundation's profile with journalists and, through them, with health and health care decision makers.

In 2008, we took another large step in supporting quality journalistic coverage of issues important to us by giving a grant to Columbia University's Graduate School of Journalism to underwrite the health and science portion of its new one-year master of arts journalism degree program. To be called the Robert Wood Johnson Foundation Program in Health and Science Journalism, it will train young and midcareer journalists to bring depth to their coverage of health and science, and provide students with specialized knowledge and a sense of context and history. The public and policymakers need reporters and editors who can effectively explain and compellingly present complex issues of health and health care.

The Foundation is coordinating with Columbia to ensure that curriculum development broadly reflects the goals and interests of the Foundation. We also will invite students to come to Princeton to meet with program and communications officers working in their fields of interest, and Robert Wood Johnson Foundation staff members will periodically travel to Columbia to speak and to provide guidance and expertise. Students in the program will become Robert Wood Johnson Foundation Fellows in Health and Science Journalism. As part of the Foundation's scholars and fellows programs, this cadre of journalists will enrich our alumni network and strengthen the Foundation's impact on the future of health and health care in this country. Not incidentally, we hope our grant also helps promote our influence with health and health care journalists.

Reach Outside Mainstream Media

Many of the key audiences and constituencies we serve—those most affected by childhood obesity and by inequities in quality of care, our most vulnerable populations, the nation's diverse group of health workers and professionals—go outside mainstream media channels for credible information. At the same time, many journalists working for media outlets serving specifically ethnic or culturally based audiences often say that health coverage is a major priority for the communities they serve. These newspaper, magazine, broadcast, and Web outlets are deeply interested in receiving culturally relevant health information from credible organizations. For many such publications and programs, their role goes beyond simply informing their audience; they also help empower people and are leading voices for change in their communities. African American and Hispanic journalists in particular often see themselves as activist participants in, rather than merely observers and reporters about, their communities. They've told us that they're interested in covering some of the Foundation's key areas of work, such as disparities, access to care, obesity, and prevention. We believe we are well positioned to provide the pipeline of information that these journalists, producers, and managers need and desire.

Serving various multicultural groups with quality health and health care information will not be an easy task. Aside from a few powerhouse entities like Univision and Spanish-language wire services, multicultural media outlets tend to be small-scale and fragmented across a wide array of ethnic subgroups and narrow geographic locations. Even so, we have supported them, both through our national program, Sound Partners for Community Health, and through a series of grants to Radio Bilingue in Fresno, California.[10]

Multicultural media journalists with whom we interact, especially at Spanish-language outlets, express a strong preference for diverse spokespeople, since the audiences for such media place greater value on hearing from experts from similar racial, ethnic, and cultural backgrounds. We currently do not have a large pool of Foundation or even grantee spokespeople to draw upon for this purpose. And there is a growing interest in data and research that is specific to multicultural audiences and their needs. In other words, they are looking for targeted news they can use from people they know, can trust, and speak their language both literally and culturally.

By focusing staff attention and resources to serve ethnic and culturally based audiences with important health information, we will significantly increase the impact of Foundation programs among key populations while also infusing the Foundation's organizational culture with the appreciation that working with diverse audiences is a default tactic, not a special project.

The days of the low Foundation profile—of hiding our light under a bushel—are gone for us because they have to be gone. We can best aid in the accomplishment of our targeted policy-change goals through speaking out directly and collaboratively, not staying in the background anymore. We are far from mastering this new on-stage role. Sometimes we are not aggressive enough in getting our messages out. Sometimes our internal processes slow us down and we miss opportunities to have an impact. Sometimes we still get tangled up with grantees who are not quite singing the same song we are. But in general we think our updating of the communications model takes us in the right direction—a direction of which Frank Karel would approve. It's a model that fits the needs and the goals of the modern Robert Wood Johnson Foundation—even if it doesn't always fit with quiet Foundation culture and our inherent modesty and wonkiness.

Notes

1. Karel, F. "Getting the Word Out: A Foundation Memoir and Personal Journey." *To Improve Health and Health Care 2001: The Robert Wood Johnson Foundation Anthology*. San Francisco: Jossey-Bass, 2001.

2. Marks, J. S. and Alper, J. "Shaping Public Policy as a Robert Wood Johnson Foundation Approach." *To Improve Health and Health Care: The Robert Wood Johnson Foundation Anthology*, Vol. XII. San Francisco: Jossey-Bass, 2009.

3. Fleishman, J. L. *The Foundation: A Great American Secret*. New York: Public Affairs, 2007.

4. *The NewsHour* and National Public Radio are grantees of the Robert Wood Johnson Foundation.

5. The Robert Wood Johnson Foundation. *2008 Assessment Report: Tracking Organizational Performance*, December 2008, http://www.rwjf.org/files/research/3632rwjf.publicscorecard081211.pdf, June 10, 2009.
6. Philanthropy Awareness Initiative. *The Challenge*, http://www.philanthropyawareness.org/challenge.php, June 10, 2009.
7. The Robert Wood Johnson Foundation. *2008 Assessment Report: Tracking Organizational Performance*.
8. The following organizations have been partners in the Covering the Uninsured campaigns: the U.S. Chamber of Commerce, AFL-CIO, Healthcare Leadership Council, AARP, United Way of America, American Medical Association, National Medical Association, American Nurses Association, Families USA, Blue Cross and Blue Shield Association, America's Health Insurance Plans, American Hospital Association, Federation of American Hospitals, Catholic Health Association of the United States, Service Employees International Union, National Alliance for Hispanic Health, The California Endowment, W. K. Kellogg Foundation, Giant Food LLC, the Kroger Co. Family of Pharmacies, Pfizer Inc., Stop & Shop, the Amateur Athletic Union, the National Association of Chain Drug Stores (NACDS).
9. Erdos & Morgan. *Opinion Leaders Study, 2008/2009, 2009*, http://www.erdosmorgan.com/sr/ols.html, June 10, 2009.
10. Diehl, D. "Sound Partners in Community Health." *To Improve Health and Health Care 2001: The Robert Wood Johnson Foundation Anthology*. San Francisco: Jossey-Bass, 2001.

CHAPTER 7

National Programs: Understanding the Robert Wood Johnson Foundation's Approach to Grantmaking

Robert G. Hughes

Editors' Introduction

Anybody trying to understand how the Robert Wood Johnson Foundation operates needs to appreciate the national program model. Since the Foundation's early years, the model has been the mainstay of the way that the Foundation develops and implements its national programs, that is, those that test ideas in a number of sites. About two-thirds of the Foundation's program expenditures have been for national programs. National program offices have traditionally provided program leadership, implementation, technical assistance, some of the Foundation's grant oversight, and communications. As Robert Hughes, a former vice president of the Foundation, notes in the reprint from Volume VIII of the *Anthology*, outsourcing these functions has allowed the Foundation to keep a relatively small staff and to involve prestigious leaders in the field in its efforts.

In 2003, the first year of Risa Lavizzo-Mourey's presidency, there were about seventy-seven national programs. Today, there are fifty-two. In some cases, functions that were previously performed by national programs have been split up and assigned to other entities, such as administrative support organizations; in other cases, they have been taken over by the Foundation itself.

The functions of the national program offices have changed since Hughes wrote this chapter in 2005. In the past, the national program director, usually a leader in the field, was the spokesperson for the program, and the national program office staff—which often included a communications director—was in charge of communications. Now the Foundation has shifted its communications strategy from one where it "speaks through its grantees" to one where it speaks for itself, as noted by Fred Mann and David Morse in Chapter 6. The new strategy has led to a strengthened central communications model based at the Foundation, and there is no longer a need to outsource this function to national programs.

Although there has been a reduction in the number of national programs, they remain an important part of the Foundation's work and are key to understanding how the Foundation and its grantees develop and implement programs.

—w—   In 1972, six people sat around a lunch table down the hall from rented offices at the former site of a nuclear accelerator in Plainsboro, New Jersey. Their wide-ranging lunchtime discussions touched on the many ways philanthropy could help improve health care and, ultimately, the health of the population. There were many such discussions among that group, all of whom were early staff members of the Robert Wood Johnson Foundation. The ideas emerging from these sessions, along with those of the Board of trustees, numerous advisers, and health care experts from around the country, shaped the basic direction of the Foundation during its formative years. Outside observers and potential grantees were most interested in what the Foundation would choose as program areas and the problems and issues that the Foundation would try to address in its grantmaking.[1] But the Foundation trustees and staff members had another question to answer—a more mundane one in some ways—how to distribute the Foundation's substantial funds responsibly.

When the Foundation received the proceeds from the estate of Robert Wood Johnson, it became the nation's second-largest philanthropy in the country overnight, with assets of more than $1 billion. The Foundation needed to award about $45 million per year. Its challenge was to make grants that would reflect Robert Wood Johnson's values and further the Board's vision for the Foundation. At the heart of the challenge was a practical administrative problem: reconciling the desire to review each grant proposal carefully and to monitor the work of each grantee with the desire to minimize the costs of this review and oversight. Underlying the practical problem were issues of control and delegation; the roles of the Board, the staff, and the grantees; and how the grantmaking mechanisms adopted would affect the Foundation's standing with its constituents.

Representing a practical compromise between the Foundation's desire to maintain a relatively small staff and minimal bureaucracy and its need to monitor programs scrupulously, a mechanism called the national program emerged as the Foundation's principal vehicle for grantmaking. In a national program, an organization outside the Foundation would oversee a set of grants related to a particular field. Experts in fields that were the focus of national programs would not have to be hired by the Foundation as employees but would remain in their home institutions, devoting a percentage of their time to the program. When the program ended, they would simply resume their former duties.

Throughout the Foundation's thirty-three-year history as a national philanthropy, national programs have been used to distribute the bulk of the Foundation's grants. Approximately 65 percent of the more than $5 billion in grants since 1972 has been awarded via 219 national programs.

—ᷫᷤ— What Is a National Program?

While no two national programs appear exactly alike, most of them have six basic characteristics in common:

1. *Foundation staff members and national experts, sometimes working with a consultant not on the Foundation's staff, develop a program designed either to address a problem of national scope or to take a promising model or idea that has received limited exposure and subject it to broader testing.* Such programs typically emerge over a year or two through a process of meetings, reviews, consultations, and revisions that involve Foundation staff members, outside experts, and practitioners from the field. During this developmental period, a program's purpose is refined, and many of its basic features—such as desired outcomes, number of grantees, grantee activities, eligibility criteria for applicant organizations, amount of grants, and duration of the program—are discussed and drafted.

2. *A call for proposals, or CFP, is distributed to potential applicants and others in the field.* The CFP defines the problems or the issues central to the program and describes the program's purpose; the desired outcomes; eligibility criteria for applicants; how the funds may be used; the criteria and the process for selecting grantees, grant amounts, and duration; and the number of grants or sites to be funded. In addition, a CFP includes the application and selection timetable, and identifies the individuals and the organizations responsible for management, oversight, and evaluation of the program. CFPs are distributed after the Board of trustees authorizes a program. Substantial changes in the program—such as major revisions of its purposes or activities, an extension of its duration, and additional funding—must be approved by the Board.

3. *Grantees are selected through a national competitive process, and any organization that meets the program's eligibility criteria can apply.* The selection of program sites—grantees under the program   from among the applicants is done by a national advisory committee, or NAC, made up of experts from a variety of areas related to the program. The NAC members review the written proposals, conduct site visits at selected applicant institutions, and recommend applicants for funding to the Foundation. The NAC is typically asked to meet periodically throughout the life of the program, providing advice and counsel to the national director of the program as well as monitoring and reporting on the progress of the program to the Foundation.

4. *The Foundation establishes a National Program Office, or NPO, external to the Foundation.* Usually based at a university or other nonprofit organization, an NPO organizes the grantee selection process and

the work of the national advisory committee. After
grantees are selected by the Foundation and funds
are awarded, an NPO monitors the work carried out
under the grant, provides technical assistance to the
program sites, and facilitates collaboration and the
sharing of information—through annual meetings,
for instance. In most cases, NPOs are expected to
provide leadership to the field. A distinctive feature
of national programs, NPOs are the Foundation's
solution to the basic administrative dilemma of
wanting knowledgeable and thorough program
oversight while at the same time avoiding an unduly
large home-office staff.

5. *Formal program evaluations, intended to help the Foundation and the field learn from national programs, are
conducted by organizations independent of the Foundation, the NPO, and the sites funded under the program.*
Selected by a competitive process, the evaluators use
social science and anthropological and other widely
accepted techniques to assess program impact, effectiveness, implementation, and other aspects of performance. Evaluators are expected to produce final
reports meeting the standards of appropriate scientific and professional journals, and are encouraged to
submit their reports for publication in peer-reviewed
and other journals and to present their findings at
professional meetings.

6. *Information about the programs is shared with the
field through communications activities.* National
programs are supposed to have an impact beyond
the sites themselves, and publicity about a program's
activities and results is essential if this is to occur.
Similarly, communications support, often from a
program's inception, is needed if the activities of
participating sites are to continue after the grant ends.
These communications functions may be carried out

by the NPO staff, by Foundation staff members, by outside consultants, or by a combination of these options.

These six characteristics make up the basic framework of the Foundation's national program model. A brief overview of more than eighty national programs operating in 2003 conveys the scale and the considerable range within this general model: the number of sites in a national program ranges from fewer than ten to several hundred, with an average of about twenty-five. Grants to program sites vary from tens of thousands to millions of dollars; the average is $300,000.

These numbers indicate the flexibility that the national program mechanism allows. Indeed, highlighting the common features of national programs may convey the idea that national program structures are straightforward and are more similar to one another than different. In fact, however, national programs vary in size and scope, and the six components are often modified to reflect a particular program's needs.

—⁓— Philanthropy and the Robert Wood Johnson Foundation in 1972

How did the Robert Wood Johnson Foundation come to develop national programs with these six basic characteristics as its principal grantmaking approach? The answer begins in 1972, when the Foundation received the endowment from the estate of Robert Wood Johnson. At that time, all of the ten largest foundations had been established for at least twenty years, and it would be twenty years more until the next cluster of new large foundations would come along. The Robert Wood Johnson Foundation might have relied on established foundations as models, but in the 1960s a series of congressional hearings critical of big philanthropies culminated in 1969 legislation establishing stricter laws to govern foundations. The hearings raised concerns about the political influence of foundations—from supporting voter-registration drives to being refuges for governmental officials who had left office. These hearings and the resulting legislation received considerable public attention, and thus sensitized Robert Wood Johnson Foundation officials to the risks that had brought controversy to other large foundations.[2]

The Foundation's initial focus on health care set it apart from other large foundations (which made grants in multiple areas, such as education, economic development, the arts, poverty, and the environment) and limited its substantive area of grantmaking. Funding only in the United States further concentrated the Foundation's grantmaking; many other large foundations made grants for international projects. Thus, the Robert Wood Johnson Foundation's domestic health care mission helped set the stage for the development of a distinctive grantmaking approach.

While the health care mission conveyed clearly what would not be funded, the task of selecting from the many worthwhile topics and problems within health care remained. By 1972, the country had come to rely on government for basic biomedical research (via the National Institutes of Health, which began to burgeon in the 1960s) and for health care financing for the elderly and the poor (via Medicare and Medicaid, begun in 1965). Counterparts to notable philanthropic health successes earlier in the century—such as Rockefeller's hookworm eradication in the South and the development of a yellow fever vaccine—would not be matched in this new era of huge government funding. Rather, a new, more selective focus within health care was needed to avoid duplication with governmental activities and to leverage the Foundation's grantmaking.[3]

The widely expected passage of national health insurance legislation during the Nixon administration provided a framework. As the very first Foundation staff paper stated, "the reconstitution of the Robert Wood Johnson Foundation as a national philanthropic organization comes at a unique point in American history. The nation has reached the culmination of a forty-year debate over the need to eliminate economic barriers to access to personal health services. Thus, within three years, we believe we are likely to see the enactment of some form of national health insurance program." National health insurance would address financing, but it also would highlight the health care system's inability to deliver care, especially primary care, for the entire population. This led the Foundation to choose improving access to primary care as one of its three initial goals.[4] The Foundation planned to reach this goal in part by demonstrating innovative models of service delivery that the federal government could adopt for the anticipated new national health care financing system. Demonstration projects in multiple locations fit well with the grantmaking mechanism of national programs.

These factors influenced the Foundation's initial grantmaking approach, but the biggest influence was a 1949 report prepared for the Ford Foundation as it coped with a similar stage in its organizational history. As Robert Wood Johnson Foundation officials talked with those at other large foundations to learn how they had structured their grantmaking, this report emerged as a seminal document. The *Report of the Study for the Ford Foundation on Policy and Program* was a wide-ranging document, the culmination of an effort that included twenty-two other special and individual reports.[5] It was prepared in anticipation of the Foundation's receiving large endowments from the estates of Henry Ford and Edsel Ford. One section of the report, "The Administration of the Program," was particularly relevant for the Robert Wood Johnson Foundation, because it presented a "suggested pattern of operations"—grantmaking approaches—for the Ford Foundation. The practical issues associated with granting large sums of money are seldom the topic of thoughtful analysis, so this was an unusual document.

The report's authors highlighted two ideas that guided their thinking in producing recommendations: maintaining flexibility of operations and giving trustees the best opportunity to guide the program in a general way. These ideas were reflected in recommendations for the types of institutions the Ford Foundation should work with and the roles of the trustees and the staff. First, the report recommended that the Ford Foundation not become involved in direct program operations but, rather, work through other organizations: These so-called intermediary organizations, which could be existing institutions such as universities or new entities established specifically to further the program's purpose, "would be free to administer the fund and make grants from it quite independently of the Foundation."

According to the Ford report, the role of the trustees was to set the general direction and to address policy questions—not to review individual grant proposals. The report pointed out that for the trustees to carry out their responsibility, they should not get involved in the detailed operations of the foundation. In keeping with the independence of intermediary organizations, the report stated, "Once a grant is given for a project, the Foundation officer should not attempt to control it. On the contrary, he should make every effort to leave full responsibility in the hands of the man in charge of the project and if asked for advice he should give it only with restraint and detachment." The staff and the trustees could review a body of work when an intermediary's term was done, with an eye toward renewal of work in that topical area, or not, depending on the merits. The report recommended recruiting a staff with a broad range of interests so that expertise in one area did not become a liability when the Foundation moved on to other areas.

In sum, the report to the Ford Foundation envisioned a structure in which the trustees would operate at a policy level (by examining broad issues, setting the foundation's direction, and judging performance); the staff would be more involved in implementation but would have sufficient detachment to make critical judgments and recommendations about the grantmaking directions and to assess the performance of intermediary organizations; and intermediaries would do most of the operational work of making and monitoring individual grants.

Many of the basic features of this proposed structure appealed to the Robert Wood Johnson Foundation. Both the Board and the early staff members wanted to maintain flexibility and did not want to develop a large staff. On the other hand, in 1972 there were strong influences on the Robert Wood Johnson Foundation to maintain tight oversight of future grantees. These influences included the public scrutiny of philanthropy in general and of a new large foundation in particular; the values of Robert Wood Johnson; and the culture of Johnson & Johnson, from whose ranks most of the early Board members came, which called for careful attention to detail and for close monitoring of budgets. So while the proposed Ford Foundation model of operations was appealing, the extent to which it ceded responsibility to intermediaries was not compatible with the heritage of the founder and the company whose stock was the source of the Foundation's endowment. It also ran against the environment of the time, which culminated in the 1969 Tax Reform Act—the act that required greater accountability and oversight on the part of private foundations.

As a result of these tensions—maintaining flexibility versus exercising control; delegating responsibility versus maintaining careful oversight; utilizing the expertise of leaders in the field versus delegating too much authority over Foundation resources—the Foundation adopted a variation on the approach recommended by the Ford Foundation report. It built on the idea of using intermediaries, but the design features were developed over time through the practical work of grantmaking.

—∿— Initial National Programs

Every year from 1972 to 1978, the Foundation initiated two to four programs that, in retrospect, can be recognized as national programs. The 1973 *Annual Report* noted that two external organizations, the National Academy of Sciences and the American Fund for Dental Education, were responsible for administering programs to establish emergency medical systems and dental care for the handicapped, respectively. The term "national program" was used only to describe the Clinical Scholars Program, which was administered by an outside director on the faculty of the University of California, San Francisco, although the use of the term was not intended at the time to denote a set of specific program characteristics. The 1974 *Annual Report* stated that the Foundation had "launched seven national programs of differing size and complexity," emphasizing several structural features: they were invitational, open to "a wider group than commonly receive foundation assistance," and used outside professional groups for formulation and design. It also noted, "In an effort to keep our internal staff small, an outside organization has often been asked to assume responsibilities for implementation and day-to-day management." The 1975 *Annual Report* listed eight national programs and contained a chart showing the amount and percentage of grants that went to these programs. It captured this constellation of characteristics in a summary description: "Foundation-initiated invitational programs—our national programs."

How did the national program model become established in just a few years? Several early programs incorporated design features that became part of the Foundation's national program model. The Board authorized the first national program, for scholarship funds at American medical and osteopathic schools, at a level of $10 million. The Association of American Medical Colleges, or AAMC, administered this program for $10,000 a year, foreshadowing the role that would become a National Program Office. "The Association has ready access to the information required, an experienced statistical staff, and first-rate management," a staff paper noted at the time. "Thus the Foundation can undertake a program involving the administration of 115 grants with minimal expenditure of the time of its own limited staff."

The Emergency Medical Services Program was the first to include a competitive call for proposals, or CFP. The CFP told the field the grant amounts ($400,000) and the number to be awarded (forty to fifty), who could apply, and the selection criteria a national advisory committee of experts from the field would use to choose grantees. The Foundation awarded a separate $300,000 grant to the National Academy of Sciences to administer the program, which included managing the advisory committee, site visits, and evaluation. In choosing an outside organization, "the Foundation is following a policy of decentralizing the administration of single-purpose national grantmaking programs of limited time duration," thus augmenting the responsibilities of an intermediary beyond what the AAMC had done in administering the student aid program.

Quickly on the heels of the Emergency Medical Services national program, three new demonstration programs—Dental Training for Care of the Handicapped, the Community Hospital–Medical Staff Group Practices Program, and the Regionalized Perinatal Care Program—reinforced the basic design features: a program developed by staff and senior program consultants, a widely publicized CFP, and the use of expert national advisory committees to review proposals and conduct site visits. However, the Foundation did not use the national program model only for demonstrations. Two programs the Foundation started funding in 1973—the Clinical Scholars Program and the Health Policy Fellows Program—illustrated the versatility of the national program model by using it for initiatives supporting leadership training for health professionals. These programs supported individuals rather than organizations providing services, but they used the basic design structure, including an external National Program Office and a national advisory committee to review applicants. The Clinical Scholars Program, which had been picked up from the Commonwealth Fund and the Carnegie Corporation of New York, already had projects at five universities, so the existing multisite idea was consistent with the developing national program model.

Evaluation has been a critical component of the national program model. But the model didn't create the institutional commitment; rather, the commitment to assess programs existed from the time the Foundation became a national philanthropy, and it was incorporated into the model. A 1973 staff paper noted, "We envision a Foundation which supports demonstration programs as proposed solutions to health problems, which provides mechanisms for evaluating these demonstrations, and through such processes, attempts to resolve those health problems that arise." The earliest national programs had evaluations built in, and as the model evolved, it became the norm for the Foundation to make a grant to an outside organization—not the NPO—for the purpose of evaluating a national program.

A final national program design element—communications—was prompted by staff thinking about what, if anything, the Foundation should do as a national program neared its conclusion. As the EMS program was ending, staff members examined options for the sustainability of existing program sites and the replication of the tested model in other sites. Replication, in particular, was a conceptual underpinning of the national program model when it was used for service demonstrations. The Foundation added communications to the national program design for two purposes: "to ensure that new options emerging from our programs gain sufficient visibility to receive appropriate consideration nationally" and "to share the knowledge, experience, and insights gained in our programs with those who decide to accept the new option and begin the process of replication."

The application of communications to foster sustainability came later. Other types of technical assistance, for grantees as well as for similar programs throughout the country, were prompted in order to help promote replication and foster the sustainability of funded projects. While technical assistance was typically provided by the National Program Office, other organizations were also used. "We have found that companion efforts can maximize the success of a national program," a 1974 staff paper noted. "For example, as part of the EMS program administered by the National Academy of Sciences organization, the Foundation and the American Medical Association are cosponsoring four workshops open to all program applicants."

The Foundation's initial grantmaking experience with unsolicited proposals from the field reinforced the value of inviting organizations to compete for grants through national programs. David Rogers, the Foundation's first president, captured this aspect of national programs in the 1974 *Annual Report*. After noting that the Foundation had made many single grants to organizations that sought help for projects within the Foundation's areas of interest, he wrote that this kind of grantmaking

> made us recognize that in a number of instances, multiple groups or institutions simultaneously wish to attack the same problem in different regions, using their particular resources, or their particular circumstances, in different, yet quite similar ways. This kind of broadly voiced interest in a particular problem has led us to develop a series of one-time grants nationally announced, and awarded in a number of institutions participating in a broader national effort directed at a particular need. These are foundation-initiated programs in areas where a certain critical level of activity seems needed to gain experience with, or demonstrate the worth of, a particular approach.

—ᘿ— Early Assessment of the National Program Approach

Aware that its behavior was closely scrutinized by Congress, staff members of the young Robert Wood Johnson Foundation thought carefully about how they did their grantmaking. Around the time that the idea of a national program coalesced, a staff paper entitled "National Competitive Grant Programs" examined the advantages and the disadvantages of such programs.

Heading the list of advantages was the fact that programs were "open to all." Early on, the Foundation decided on a process open to a wide variety of applicants. "We made these decisions with the belief that the difficulties many groups have obtaining information about and access to grants has been the Achilles' heel of foundations, and it has caused many to feel that foundations are elitist or arbitrary in their awards," David Rogers and two of his senior Foundation colleagues wrote in 1983. "Because of unfamiliarity with foundations in general, or a lack of understanding of our mission in particular, many who might make important contributions to the improvement of health affairs might not find their way to us unless we make a special effort to reach out to a broad constituency."[6] The Foundation valued the fairness and the benefits of a competitive process based on expert judgments and clear criteria. This process was an antidote to the reality and the perception that it was an insider's game in which who you knew was more important than demonstrated merit or promise. It also reduced the risk that the Robert Wood Johnson Foundation would be criticized for perceived political bias in its grantmaking practices.

This open competition was compatible with the emphasis on the "national" in national program. For Board members, a national perspective was important as a way of distinguishing the post-1972 Foundation from the earlier Robert Wood Johnson Foundation, with its focus on central New Jersey. In fact, the Robert Wood Johnson Foundation's first letter to potential applicants said that it would concentrate on programs that were "fully national in scope" and that it would support those that showed "promise of having significant regional and national impact."[7]

A national perspective was also important in its geographic sense. Annual reports typically included a chart showing percentage of grants, dollars, and American population for each region of the country to demonstrate that the Foundation's activities were widely distributed (and, implicitly, that they were not bundled locally as a result of favoritism). An anecdote, perhaps apocryphal, indicates how valuable this distribution was to Gustav Lienhard, chairman of the Board from 1972 to 1985. A conference room had a United States map displayed with pins to indicate the location of early Foundation grants. After looking at this map one day and seeing a concentration of pins in the Northeast, Lienhard said, "Scatter the pins!"—an admonition that has shaped Foundation grantmaking ever since. This approach, which supported a large number of local projects nationwide, also satisfied Board members who valued a traditional charity program that helped people, while accommodating those who valued the analysis and evaluation activities that contributed to useful knowledge about program effectiveness.

Moreover, the national program model was valued for its efficiency. "The development of a national program is a time-consuming process, but probably modest in contrast to the considerable time and resources that are expended by the Foundation staff in developing a single proposal," an early staff paper noted.

While a national program approach using a competitive grant application process had great advantages for the fledgling Foundation, it did not answer the question of whether programs should be overseen from inside or outside the Foundation—the very question raised by the 1949 report to the Ford Foundation. An analysis of the pros and cons of using external National Program Offices to administer grants identified the several advantages and disadvantages as shown in Table 7.1.

Table 7.1.   Advantages and Disadvantages of Using External Program Offices to Administer Grants

Advantages	Disadvantages
Keeps headquarters staff small	Less control over programs
Permits Foundation staff to plan longer range	If poorly administered by partner, considerable Princeton staff time required
Removes the Foundation from basic selection process—reduces criticism and places pressure directly on Princeton staff	Partner organization may have different perception of its role from that of the Foundation
Involves a major organization as a partner with the Foundation—which should enhance the Foundation's prestige	Key executive officer of partner organization may have different perception of his role than the Foundation
Educational for the Foundation—partner organization will learn things from the field that the staff would not	Complicated to administer

The list suggests the underlying issues at play. The desire to keep the staff small was pitted against the risk of losing control over program administration. Inconsistencies between the Foundation's view of a program and a partner organization's view could create conflicts. The division of responsibility between the Foundation and an outside institution was ambiguous. But one design feature not mentioned was unambiguous—who controlled the money, and that was the Foundation. The outside institution received its own grant, of course, but the program sites were funded directly by the Foundation, not through the partner organization. Accordingly, advice from national advisory committees about which applicants to fund went to the Foundation, not to the National Program Office. This role for NPOs was considerably less than the intermediary role recommended in the Ford Foundation report. The decision to retain fiscal oversight by the Foundation was a critical one that has shaped the roles, responsibilities, and relationships of Foundation staff members, NPOs, and program grantees ever since.

In addition to the substantive and administrative issues, the emergence of national programs had a political dimension. The national program model afforded considerable credibility to a new foundation. As a new entity, the Robert Wood Johnson Foundation had an uncertain standing in philanthropy and in health care. The Foundation gained immediate prestige when the Board of trustees selected David Rogers, dean of the Johns Hopkins School of Medicine, as the Foundation's president. The recruitment of experienced staff members from other foundations also gave the Foundation credibility in the philanthropic community. Within the health care community, the national program model helped the young Foundation establish credibility because it engaged health care experts in all facets of the program, especially as leaders of National Program Offices, as members of national advisory committees, and as senior program consultants.

Many National Program Offices and grantees were also part of the Foundation's primary constituency—academic health centers and medical schools in particular. Indeed, in the Foundation's first three years, 65 percent of the funds went to academic centers.[8] The national program model was compatible with the way academic health centers operated. They relied extensively on grants; faculties cooperated across institutions in multisite clinical trials and other research projects; they were accustomed to a competitive peer-review system of grant selection; and the intermingling of practice with science in medicine paralleled the combination of demonstration with evaluation in Foundation programs.

—⌇— Evolution of National Programs

As a grantmaking vehicle, the national program mechanism has been remarkably consistent since it was established in the mid-1970s. The basic structure has become institutionalized within the Robert Wood Johnson Foundation. A 2003 national program such as Active Living by Design, which integrates physical activity into community planning efforts, looks, in its grantmaking structure, remarkably similar to the Emergency Medical Systems Program, launched thirty years earlier. But this consistency in basic structure should not obscure two important aspects of the evolution of national programs: the increasing number of programs and the variations within the basic model.

The increasing number of national programs—the Foundation had more than eighty in 2004—was driven by five interrelated factors: growth in Foundation assets and staff, staff incentives, increased diversity of funding areas, decreased size of programs, and the continuation of existing programs, even as new ones were added. As Foundation assets have grown over the years, new staff members have been hired to oversee the concomitant increase in grants. For Foundation staff members, developing a national program became a hallmark accomplishment; it was one of the few ways a program officer could gain recognition within the Foundation and in the field generally. Over the past thirty-plus years, the Foundation has entered new substantive areas—tobacco control and end-of-life care, for instance—and this has required new programs with new institutions and people. The pressures for new programs led ineluctably to smaller programs, although this was not obvious because the nominal size of national programs remained fairly constant, at around $10 million. But $10 million in 1973 dollars was approximately $40 million in 2003, so in real dollars the programs became smaller. Finally, as existing programs were renewed while new programs were developed, the net result was an increasing number of active programs.

The second important aspect of the evolution of national programs was the variation among NPOs.

- The types of organizations used as NPOs have been diverse: professional associations, medical care delivery organizations, independent nonprofit entities, and policy institutes joined academic institutions as NPOs.

- The staffing of NPOs became less standard—some had full-time program directors, communications staff, and financial monitoring staff; deputy directors, who formerly were responsible for standard administrative functions, assumed more prominence, and in some cases were virtually indistinguishable from the directors in their substantive contributions to the field.

- NPOs have played a variety of roles. Some NPOs, such as the Center for Health and Health Care in Schools at George Washington University and Join Together, are resource centers that provide technical assistance to organizations in their fields across the country. The Center for Prevention Research at the University of Kentucky, the NPO for the Research Network on the Etiology of Tobacco Dependence, administers a network program structure that fosters intellectual work among grantees. Several NPOs experimented with new grantmaking roles—for example, by administering special grant funds for projects to take advantage of fast-breaking opportunities. A few NPOs, such as the Center for Health Care Strategies, which is the NPO for the Medicaid Managed Care Program, took on direct responsibility for grantee selection under the program, moving closer to a more independent intermediary role.

The evolution of national program structures is reflected in their nomenclature and brief descriptions found in the Foundation's annual reports. Table 7.2 lists these for 1973–2002.

Initially, only the names and the degrees of the senior program consultants were listed; the job title changed to "program director" in 1988. This original listing emphasized a person rather than an organization, and that person was considered an expert with a consulting relationship to the Foundation (even when the consultant's home institution had a grant to administer the program). Defining that person as a consultant reinforced the Foundation's authority over the program. The shift to "program director" in 1993 connoted that the program's leader shared responsibility for the program with the Foundation, an idea that was strengthened by adding "National Program Office" to the heading. Contact information for the NPO was included for the first time, along with an explanation that stated, "Most of these

Table 7.2. National Programs, 1973–2002

Date	Title	Information	No. of NPs
1973–1987	Senior Program Consultants	Name, degree	4–24
1988–1992	Program Directors	Name, degree	24–37
1993–2000	National Program Offices and National Program Directors	Program name Director's name Organization and address	37–80
2001–2003	National Program Offices and Resource Centers	Program name Organization and address Website address Director's name and e-mail address	80

programs are managed by institutions outside the Foundation." The most recent change, in the 2001 *Annual Report*, emphasized the growing heterogeneity of program structures and associated strategies by referring to intermediary organizations as "National Program Offices and Resource Centers."

The quantity and the variety of national programs have produced administrative challenges for the Foundation. The large number of small programs increased the staff needed to develop, monitor, and learn from individual programs. The variety of program models has resulted in ambiguity and duplication of roles between Foundation staff and NPO staff. This is costly and erodes the benefits of delegation to outside offices. Growing recognition of these issues led to an October 2003 staff paper that reviewed the Foundation's use of NPOs. Based on an internal study of National Program Offices as a vehicle for grantmaking and grant management, the staff paper found that using so many different NPOs to perform common functions led to "inefficiencies." The paper focused on the same question raised in the report to the Ford Foundation's Board back in 1949—which functions should be performed internally by the Foundation's staff and which should be delegated to outside organizations.

The answers are still not in, and the Robert Wood Johnson Foundation is still looking for the appropriate balance between in-house and external program management. In the current environment, where nonprofit organizations must be more accountable, foundations must devote appropriate resources not only to making grants but also to monitoring programs, assessing performance, learning what works, and communicating with the field and the public. To meet the challenges, the Foundation needs to identify clearly the variety of program models it will use, so that staff and grantees alike understand their roles in the program model they work within. Equally important, to increase the overall effectiveness of its programs, the Foundation needs to learn how different program models relate to the impact of the programs.

—ᴍ— Conclusions

National programs as a grantmaking approach emerged as a compromise between the delegation of grantmaking responsibility to an intermediary organization and retaining the responsibility within the Foundation. The benefits of delegation (avoiding a foundation bureaucracy, flexibility, use of outside experts, and a staff focus on learning from investments rather than spending time on the mechanics of retail grantmaking) were at odds with the benefits of maintaining direct control over the use of Foundation grants (specifying program goals and activities, understanding grantees' work, and holding grantees accountable financially and programmatically). The hybrid that developed had the benefits of both approaches, but it also had their disadvantages. Almost inevitably, the insistence on control and detailed plans for the use of grant funds required staff growth within the Foundation and an emphasis on grantmaking over learning about the results of multiple investments in a program area. At the same time, partial delegation of program responsibilities has resulted in inefficiencies and confusion about the relative roles of Foundation and National Program Office staff. The future challenge for national program design is to use grantmaking approaches that exploit the advantages and minimize the disadvantages of both approaches.

Notes

1. Farber, M. "Suddenly Wealthy Johnson Foundation Maps Plans." *New York Times*, May 12, 1972.
2. Gardner, JR. and Harrison AR. "The Robert Wood Johnson Foundation: The Early Years," *To Improve Health and Health Care Volume VIII*. San Francisco: Jossey-Bass, 2005.
3. Blendon, R. "The Changing Role of Private Philanthropy in Health Affairs." *New England Journal of Medicine*, 1975, *292*, 946–950.
4. The other two initial goals were improving the quality of health and medical care and developing mechanisms for objective analysis of public policies in health. *The Robert Wood Johnson Foundation Annual Report*. Princeton, NJ: Robert Wood Johnson Foundation, 1972.

5. Study Committee (H. R. Gaither Jr., chairman). "Report of the Study for the Ford Foundation on Policy and Program." Ford Foundation, November 1949.
6. Blendon, R., Aiken, L., and Rogers, D. "Improving Health and Medical Care in the United States: A Foundation's Early Experience." *Journal of Ambulatory Care Management*, November 1983, 1–11.
7. "Information on the Robert Wood Johnson Foundation." Informational letter to all applicants, September 25, 1972.
8. *Chartbook of Expenditures 1972–1974*. Princeton, NJ: Robert Wood Johnson Foundation, 1975.

Thanks to the many people who have shared their understanding of national programs with me. In particular, Calvin Bland, Peter Goodwin, Ruby Hearn, Rona Henry, Frank Karel, Terry Keenan, Julia Lear, Janice Opalski, and Warren Wood helped develop my understanding of national programs. Bob Blendon, who by all accounts was a principal architect of the national program model, was especially helpful in articulating the impact of the Ford Foundation Report on the Foundation's thinking early on. Special thanks to Andrew Harrison for assistance in locating Foundation historical material. Of course, I remain ultimately responsible for the ideas expressed in this chapter.

CHAPTER 8

Tending Our Backyard: The Robert Wood Johnson Foundation's Grantmaking in New Jersey

Pamela S. Dickson

Editors' Introduction

In Volume V of the *Anthology*, Pamela Dickson, then a senior program officer at the Foundation and now the assistant vice president for health care, wrote that the Robert Wood Johnson Foundation has funded programs and people in the New Brunswick area and throughout New Jersey "in part to honor the legacy of its founder, and in part to recognize the special responsibilities to the communities and the state in which it is located." In the decade since "Tending Our Backyard: The Robert Wood Johnson Foundation's Grantmaking in New Jersey" was published, the Foundation has maintained its charitable giving in New Jersey, but has adjusted it so that it is more strategically focused on important health issues.

Perhaps the clearest example of this reorientation is the New Jersey Health Initiatives. In the past, the New Jersey Health Initiatives had issued a yearly call for proposals for projects falling generally within the Foundation's priorities.

Now it issues annual calls for proposals for a number of projects focused on a single theme. To date, these include projects designed to:

- Address behavioral issues confronting young men who are at risk for substance abuse, gang involvement, and dropping out of school

- Improve patients' transitions of care from one facility to another (for example, from a hospital to a nursing home)

- Develop community needs assessments and implement health improvement plans through collaborations among hospitals, health departments, and other community agencies

- Build the capacity of community-based organizations serving vulnerable population groups, including members of historically underrepresented groups and low-income individuals

- Combat teen dating violence

- Strengthen the health literacy of new immigrants

Furthermore, New Jersey Health Initiatives selectively replicates in the state programs that have shown promise nationally, such as Expecting Success, a program aimed at improving the overall quality of cardiac care while reducing racial, ethnic, and language disparities. Another national program, Reclaiming Futures, which seeks to improve the way the juvenile justice system handles young people with substance abuse problems, is currently under consideration as a program to be replicated in New Jersey.

Beyond the New Jersey Health Initiatives, the Foundation is developing programs in New Jersey that fall within its national priority areas—such as childhood obesity. The New Jersey Partnership for Healthy Kids is working to reduce childhood obesity by improving nutrition and increasing physical activity among children living in five communities: Camden, Newark, New Brunswick, Trenton, and Vineland. The Foundation is also funding the establishment of the New Jersey Institute for Food, Nutrition, and Health at Rutgers University's New Brunswick campus. And through a $10 million loan and a $2 million grant (with additional support from the New Jersey Economic Development Authority and Living Cities), the Foundation is providing the New Jersey Food Access Initiative with money to finance the establishment of twelve supermarkets in low-income communities over the next ten years.

The second priority area is nursing. The Foundation is collaborating with the state's Chamber of Commerce on the New Jersey Nursing Initiative, which directly targets the nursing shortage in New Jersey. One reason for the shortage is a lack of qualified faculty able to teach the many people who want to become nurses. The initiative provides scholarships for master's and doctoral level nursing students who can then go on to become faculty members in the state's nursing schools.

Shortly after Dickson wrote her chapter in 2001, the Foundation authorized a program to improve the health and well-being of children from birth to age three in Trenton, the state's capital—a city of roughly eighty-five thousand people that is characterized by high levels of poverty.[1] Called Children's Futures, the program serves as both an intermediary—receiving and re-granting funds to organizations providing services to very young children and their families—and as a coordinator—working with agencies and organizations providing early childhood health and social services in Trenton. In the ensuing eleven years, Children's Futures has:

- Financed home-visitation programs (that is, programs in which nurses or other health professionals visit pregnant women in their homes and provide child-rearing guidance before and after the child is born)[2]
- Funded technical assistance to child-care centers and family-child centers
- Supported a model (developed by the New Jersey Chapter of the American Academy of Pediatrics) for improving preventive care (the model was adopted by eleven of thirteen pediatric and family practices in Trenton, serving 90 percent of the city's children)
- Developed a collaborative of city agencies designed to involve fathers in their children's upbringing

Unlike its other programming, in New Jersey the Foundation will cover the cost of capital construction and economic development and will provide core support to institutions. Hence, it has made grants or loans to build and support the Cancer Institute of New Jersey, the Child Health Institute of New Jersey, and The Cardiovascular Institute of New Jersey (all at the University of Medicine and Dentistry of New Jersey); the College of Nursing and the New Jersey Institute for Food, Health, and Nutrition (both at Rutgers); and the Robert Wood Johnson University Hospital. The Foundation's support of the New Brunswick Development Corporation has helped revitalize the city.

Notes

1. The Foundation awarded $20 million in 2002 to cover 2002–2006 and an additional $14.5 million in 2006 to take the program through 2012.
2. The New Jersey home visiting program is modeled on a program developed by David Olds, whom the Foundation supported from 1979 through 2007. New Jersey is one of several states that are funding nurse home visiting programs.

—ɯ— In 1972, the Robert Wood Johnson Foundation became a philanthropy with a national mission to improve the health and health care of all Americans. It was not, however, the birth of the foundation bearing the name of Robert Wood Johnson. The chairman and chief executive officer of Johnson & Johnson created his foundation in 1936 as a vehicle for his philanthropic endeavors in the New Brunswick area, where the company's headquarters were located.

While the Robert Wood Johnson Foundation has functioned on a national scale for thirty years, in this time it also has continued funding programs and people in the New Brunswick area and throughout New Jersey. It does so in part to honor the legacy of its founder, and in part to recognize the special responsibilities to the communities and the state in which it is located.

Every national foundation, and many foundations with a statewide focus, must balance local grantmaking with broader aims. This balancing act raises, at the outset, the question of how much should be spent locally. Other questions follow logically: What criteria should be used in deciding whom and what to fund? How closely should a foundation's overall goals guide local grantmaking? Who should make local funding decisions? How can the staff effectively manage local pressures?

—ɯ— The Early Years

Robert Wood Johnson (1893–1968), the son and nephew of the cofounders of the medical products giant Johnson & Johnson, grew up in an era when wealthy individuals were expected to give back a certain portion of their wealth to the community, most typically in the form of charitable assistance to the needy. Johnson began his career as a factory worker for the company at the age of eighteen and spent his entire professional life with Johnson & Johnson. He became the president in 1932 and chairman of the Board in 1938. While Johnson was noted at an early age for his generosity and loyalty to his home town of New Brunswick, the institutional vehicle for his gift giving was the Johnson New Brunswick Foundation, which he created in 1936 with a donation of 12,000 shares of Johnson & Johnson stock and 130 acres of land along the Raritan River in New Brunswick. The Johnson New Brunswick Foundation was guided by a small Board composed of local businessmen (including Johnson & Johnson executives), but decision making appears to have remained squarely in Johnson's hands.[1]

The first award made by the Johnson New Brunswick Foundation was the deeding of 130 acres to the township of New Brunswick for a public park, later to be named Johnson Park. More typically, the Foundation's earliest grants were made to those down on their luck. Gifts ranged from food and clothing for poor families, to fixing an orphan boy's teeth before he departed for Boy's Town in Nebraska, to a down payment on a house for a highly regarded black policeman with a wife and eight children.

Two early grantees of the Johnson New Brunswick Foundation that remain connected to the Robert Wood Johnson Foundation to this day are Cenacle House and the Salvation Army. The residence that eventually became the retreat for the nuns of the Society of Our Lady of the Cenacle was originally the Johnson summer home, on a hilltop overlooking the Raritan River and New Brunswick. The Johnson Foundation donated the house and the grounds to the two daughters of James McGarry when they joined this order. McGarry had been a Johnson & Johnson mill superintendent who had befriended and taught Johnson the ropes in his first days with the company.

Brigadier General Henry Dries, who ran the operation of the Salvation Army in New Brunswick, recalled his first "grant proposal" by saying, "I first sought his [Johnson's] help to purchase the Hebrew Ladies' Aid Society building to house transients when they traveled between New York and Philadelphia. They were homeless, but we didn't call them that then. They were 'transients' and often alcoholics. Mr. Johnson didn't like the term 'alcoholic,' and he referred to them as 'men with drinking problems.'"[2] Despite the wide range of charitable endeavors funded by the Johnson New Brunswick Foundation, the most identifiable theme was support for the health care delivery system. Johnson cultivated an early and abiding involvement with hospital operations. He devoted funds and offered advice to the two general hospitals in New Brunswick: Middlesex General Hospital (now the Robert Wood Johnson University Hospital), where he chaired the executive committee for six years, and St. Peter's Hospital (now St. Peter's University Hospital). The Johnson New Brunswick Foundation supported the health care professions as well, making loans so that young men from New Brunswick could go to medical school, and sponsoring programs to elevate the professional status of nurses.

In 1952, the foundation was renamed the Robert Wood Johnson Foundation. Although this name change removed the reference to New Brunswick, the foundation continued to operate locally throughout Johnson's lifetime. Johnson continued to make regular contributions of Johnson & Johnson common stock. When he died, in 1968, the Foundation held 569,130 shares, with a value of $60,000,000.

—⚹— Outgrowing New Brunswick

Johnson left the bulk of his estate, consisting of Johnson & Johnson stock then valued at $300 million, to the Foundation. By the time probate was concluded, in 1971, the value of the shares had increased fourfold, to $1.2 billion.

Johnson did not stipulate a focus for these funds other than a general hope that they would benefit mankind. There are no minutes that reflect the trustees' decision to promote the betterment of the health of the American people, but it seems an obvious choice, in the light of Johnson's business and personal interests over his lifetime. Given the size of the assets, the trustees decided that the Foundation should assume a national presence.

The Foundation's first chairman was Gustav Lienhard, who was at the time president of Johnson & Johnson. Lienhard, who served as the Foundation's chairman and CEO until 1986, exerted great influence over the Foundation's early development, broadening its reach well beyond New Brunswick and New Jersey. He also stressed a businesslike attitude toward grantmaking, indicating a preference for sustainability and replicability in projects funded by the Foundation. Lienhard and the new Board also underscored the Foundation's focus on health by selecting as its first president Dr. David E. Rogers, the dean of the Johns Hopkins University School of Medicine. Rogers selected a program staff with national expertise in various health policy fields and developed a series of demonstration projects with sites throughout the nation.

In the *1972 Annual Report*, Rogers laid out a seventeen-page analysis of health care opportunities and strategies, and identified three national program strategies for the Foundation:

- Improving access to medical care for underserved Americans
- Improving the quality of health and medical care
- Developing mechanisms for objective analysis of public policies in health

The staff was asked to develop program priorities that would achieve these goals, and the Foundation developed a new model of grantmaking for its national programs—one that identified, in advance, a program's goals and criteria for grantee selection. This was very different from the approach used by most national foundations at the time, which tended to respond to unsolicited proposals for funds.

Even as this national perspective was being developed, local institutions saw the increase in the Foundation's assets as an opportunity to receive even more support than in the past. Recalling Johnson's generosity and anticipating the Foundation's help in purchasing land, new equipment, and other capital expansions, New Brunswick hospitals and other health care institutions made plans for capital improvements.

In the early days, the biggest challenge facing the young Foundation was meeting the new 7 percent payout required by the Tax Reform Act of 1969 (later reduced to 5 percent). As a result of the large payout requirement, little competition for resources emerged initially. Although tensions about whether to allocate funds locally or nationally surfaced occasionally in meetings of the board of trustees throughout the 1970s and 1980s, the board did not appear to have adopted a formal position on the matter. Requests for local funding were presented, reviewed, and funded on an informal basis.

The necessity of dealing with this issue came to a head, however, in the late 1980s, when the staff decided to take another look at what seemed like a continuous list of requests from Middlesex General Hospital. Once the small project budgets were aggregated, the total came to $10 million. Given the level of funding requested, the Board decided to develop a more formal policy and process to guide its central New Jersey giving. In 1990, the Board adopted a resolution that central New Jersey grants "remain at 3 percent of the Foundation's total annual grantmaking, as calculated on a five-year average." The 3 percent figure was adopted as a continuation of past trends, and was seen as more of a target than a cap. However, the Foundation's giving to local charities that reflected Robert Wood Johnson's legacy from the 1930s were considered above and beyond the 3 percent target.

—ᴡ— The Foundation's New Jersey Funding

Decisions about how much to allocate to local versus national programs, for what purposes, and how to do so reflect a complicated history and an interplay of dynamic forces ranging from the founders' wishes to the degree of specificity with which the Foundation defines its goals and the successes or failures of past grantmaking. The Robert Wood Johnson Foundation's current New Jersey funding can be sorted into four different categories:

- *Legacy Grants* are, in general, charitable donations to organizations in the New Brunswick area that were supported by, or similar to those supported by, Johnson before the Robert Wood Johnson Foundation adopted a national perspective.

- *Out-of-Program* grants are made to New Jersey organizations, predominantly in the New Brunswick area, for programs that are generally consistent with the Foundation's goals but do not necessarily fall within its priorities.

- *In-Program* grants are expected to meet the Foundation's overall goals and more specific programming priorities. These grants are earmarked for New Jersey organizations that compete only with other New Jersey applicants.

- *National Program Grants* are made to New Jersey applicants that successfully compete with other applicants throughout the nation.

Legacy Grants

Giving to New Brunswick charities, a valued tradition for the Foundation's Board, is seen as a way of honoring the Foundation's founder. Programs funded as legacy grants do not have to fall within the Foundation's mandate, nor do they go through a competitive selection process. In this regard, they are akin to the charitable donations of a community foundation. Legacy grants fund the same New Brunswick charities that were supported by Robert Wood Johnson in his early days as a philanthropist, as well as other local groups carrying out similar charitable endeavors. The Salvation Army, the Society of St. Vincent de Paul, Cenacle Retreat House, the United Way of Central New Jersey, the Plainsboro Rescue Squad and Plainsboro Volunteer

Fire Company No. 1 (the Foundation's headquarters are in Plainsboro Township), and Kiddie Keep Well Camp (a summer camp available to children with severe illness or disabilities) are among the organizations that the Robert Wood Johnson Foundation has supported for many years.

New Brunswick went through a very difficult economic period in the 1970s; it rebounded in the 1990s, and has become a thriving city. Part of the recovery can be credited to Johnson & Johnson's decision to maintain its headquarters in the city, and part can also be given to the ongoing support of the Robert Wood Johnson Foundation. The Foundation has given core support to two municipal organizations: New Brunswick Tomorrow, a network of human service agencies, and the New Brunswick Development Corporation, charged with rebuilding the downtown area.

For the most part, these grantees are sustained with annual increases adjusted for the cost of living. Funding in this category throughout the 1990s was approximately $14 million.

Table 8.1.   Selected Legacy Grants

Grantee	Year Funded	2000 Funding
Cenacle Retreat House	1949	$72,000
Salvation Army	1972	$250,000
Kiddie Keep Well Camp	1975	$322,000
New Brunswick Development Corporation	1981	$300,000
New Brunswick Tomorrow	1977	$350,000
United Way of Central Jersey	1976	$550,000
Society of St. Vincent de Paul	1972	$132,000

Out-of-Program Grants

Under the 1990 Board resolution, out-of-program grants are targeted at 3 percent of the Foundation's annual grant giving. Like legacy grants, out-of-program awards do not have to fall within the Foundation's strategic priorities. But unlike the legacy grants, which tend to be small and sustained with small increments over many years, out-of-program grants tend to be large one-time awards, even when they are made to beneficiaries that were early recipients of Johnson's largesse. Although it's not a requirement that out-of-program grants be related to health care, they tend to be so; they are typically awarded to central New Jersey health care organizations. This category of grants, together with the legacy grants, comes closest to fulfilling the Foundation's role as a good corporate neighbor. Out-of-program grants reflect a sense of pride in the state of New Jersey and an acknowledgment of its importance in the lives of Robert Wood Johnson, Johnson & Johnson, and most of the early trustees.

Many of the Foundation's out-of-program grants have gone to increase the capacity of New Jersey's health care institutions, so that the state's residents could have access to first-rate medical facilities without having to go to New York City or Philadelphia. In its earlier days, the Foundation focused on strengthening the University of Medicine and Dentistry of New Jersey, which had its headquarters in Newark and teaching sites in New Brunswick and Camden, and supporting other health care providers in Middlesex County, like the Robert Wood Johnson, Jr., Rehabilitation Institute. More recently, the Foundation made major capital gifts to help establish the New Jersey Cancer Center, the New Jersey Cardiovascular Institute, and a new Child Health Institute, all of which are in New Brunswick.

Another out-of-program grant established the Center for State Health Policy at Rutgers University in 1999. The Center aims at serving the state in two ways. First, it focuses Rutgers' academic resources on health policy development, giving it the potential to become a nationally recognized institution in this field. Second, it provides advice—based on the university's health-related expertise across a range of disciplines—to the state government. To increase the usefulness of this function, the Center brings together teams of researchers and subject-matter specialists able to respond quickly to requests from state health care decision makers for background information, research findings, and policy analyses.

Table 8.2.   Selected Out-of-Program Grants

Grantee	Year Funded	Amount
New Jersey Cardiovascular Institute	2001	$10,000,000
Child Health Institute of New Jersey	1998	$5,500,000
	2001	$10,000,000
Cancer Institute of New Jersey	1999	$6,000,000
	2001	$10,000,000
Center for State Health Policy at Rutgers	1998	$11,000,000

During the 1990s, $64 million was approved for projects in this category.

In-Program Grants

In-Program Grants occupy a middle ground between the Foundation's legacy and out-of-program grants—with their comparatively informal review process—and its national program grants—with their rigorous selection process. In-program grants are made only to New Jersey organizations for activities that fall within the priorities of the Foundation.

The rationale for creating a middle ground that gives preferential treatment to home state applicants is threefold. First, if good ideas are being put into practice elsewhere, then the Foundation ought to be sure that New Jersey also benefits. Second, such grants encourage the testing of innovative ideas in the Foundation's home state. Third, they help build health and health care expertise in New Jersey.

As the young Robert Wood Johnson Foundation began to roll out its large national programs in the 1970s, a highly competitive and rigorous process developed in which a large number of applicants would submit proposals in response to a Call for Proposals. Often, New Jersey applicants were not successful in securing grants. However, the Foundation liked the idea of including a New Jersey site when it made awards in its nationwide programs, and, as a result, it became common practice to add a New Jersey site when the successful applicant pool did not include a New Jersey organization. Eventually, the Foundation chose another route that would give preference to organizations within its home state: the New Jersey Health Initiatives.

The initial proposal to establish the New Jersey Health Initiatives, submitted to the board of trustees in December of 1986, requested the authorization of funds for "a visible effort providing seed-money grants for unusual health care innovations" within the state. It expressed the hope that the program would create an impetus for New Jersey institutions to move more rapidly in health and health care, and would provide a mechanism for assessing many of the proposals the Foundation routinely received from institutions around the state.

Under the New Jersey Health Initiatives, organizations across the state have an opportunity to respond to Calls for Proposals, issued once or twice a year, that solicit innovative community-based projects addressing one or more of the Foundation's goal areas—currently, increasing access to care, improving prevention and treatment of chronic illness, promoting healthy communities and lifestyles, and reducing the harm caused by substance abuse. The Foundation will fund grants up to $500,000 over a three-year period.

As it often does with national programs, the Robert Wood Johnson Foundation designated an outside organization to

Table 8.3.   Selected In-Program New Jersey Grants

Grantee	Year Funded	Amount
Alliance of Community Health Plans—Tobacco control in physician networks	2000	$475,000
Foundation at New Jersey Institute of Technology—Videotape for parents of disabled children	2000	$181,000
New Jersey Health Policy Forums	2000	$649,000
Caucus Education Corporation—Health care series on public television	1999	$151,000
New Jersey Minority Health Summit	1999	$50,000

administer the New Jersey Health Initiatives. Not only does this reduce the Foundation's administrative burden and tap into expertise beyond the Foundation's walls, but it also reduces the pressure on the staff from local applicants.

The first program office, beginning in January of 1987, was the Health Corporation of the Archdiocese of Newark. In the mid-1990s, the program office shifted to the Health Research and Educational Trust of New Jersey in Princeton. In 2001, the program home changed once again to the Institute for Health, Health Care Policy and Aging Research at Rutgers University. In each of its various homes, the New Jersey Health Initiatives staff manages the process in conjunction with an outside review committee. This process includes proposal review, selection of grantees, and grant administration. With the help of the advisory committee, the staff recommends to the Foundation the best candidates out of each pool for funding.

Some New Jersey Health Initiatives projects have been noteworthy. The Monmouth Medical Center, for example, organized interdisciplinary teams of medical and social service professionals to coordinate services for dying patients. The project was favorably received by patients' families, and the hospital staff was so enthusiastic that the hospital arranged relief time for staff members who wanted to participate. It became a model that the Foundation used as it was developing strategies to improve palliative care for dying patients. Another example is the New Jersey SEED Project, which supported the development of ethics training to facilitate dispute resolution in nursing homes. Although the state of New Jersey funds regional long-term-care ethics committees that offer general guidance, their resources are insufficient to provide guidance on the specific issues that arise in the care of individuals in nursing homes. The grant enabled in-house training to be made available to the staffs of many New Jersey long-term care facilities.

In addition to the New Jersey Health Initiatives, the Foundation also funds unsolicited proposals that have the potential for local impact. An example is the Capitol Policy Forums project.

Early in the 1990s, the League of Women Voters of New Jersey requested the Foundation's financial support in an effort to promote a more civil discourse on important health policy issues in New Jersey. In response, the Foundation agreed to fund a series of quarterly forums on key health issues, sponsored by the League of Women Voters of New Jersey and attended by state public policymakers and stakeholders. The Foundation continues to support these forums, now sponsored by the Forums Institute for Public Policy, and has financed similar efforts in other states.

The Foundation has also undertaken several initiatives with the New Jersey state government. In the 1980s, it contributed to the state's establishment of seven hospital consortia to transfer pregnant women with potentially high-risk deliveries to hospitals best prepared to care for endangered newborns. The funding for these consortiums has been picked up by member hospitals, and they remain in operation today.

In response to a request from the state government, the Foundation funded, between 1996 and 2000, an innovative way to monitor quality of care in nursing homes. The traditional approach involved facility inspections based largely on physical plant standards and staffing levels. However, these criteria did not measure actual resident outcomes. In the mid-1990s, the federal Health Care Financing Administration was beginning the process of creating quality-of-care indicators for nursing home residents that could be reported in an electronic format. New Jersey proposed that the new federal electronic database also be used by its state inspectors—not in a punitive way but to help nursing homes set quality-of-care goals for themselves.

The Foundation has also funded capacity-building projects in the state government. Len Fishman, Commissioner of Health from 1993 through 1998, relates that he was thrilled with the flexibility of a $50,000 award from the Foundation to be used on a health policy issue of his choosing. Later in his term, a Foundation grant enabled the Department of Health and two other state agencies to carry out a comprehensive planning process based on consolidating into a single agency all of the state's services to the elderly. That funding "brought many more people to the table than would otherwise have been possible," observed Fishman.

Over the decade of the 1990s, the Foundation made 286 in-program New Jersey grants totaling $86 million.

National Program Grants

New Jersey organizations, like those from any other state, can respond to Calls for Proposals and seek funds for national programs in areas identified as priorities by the Robert Wood Johnson Foundation. New Jersey applicants receive no special advantages in these competitions, and, like applicants from any state, face tough odds in them. There are, however, some outstanding examples of New Jersey grantees having competed successfully. For example, the New Jersey Breathes project, run by the New Jersey Medical Society, was one of the original nine sites in the SmokeLess States program. New Jersey Breathes and its partners in the state engaged in public education about the harmful impact of cigarette smoking among young people. The issue received widespread attention, and, in 1997, the state cigarette tax was increased.

—∿— Conclusion

As currently structured, the Foundation's New Jersey grantmaking maintains certain of its central values, principally by honoring its founder, serving as a corporate good neighbor, standing behind grantees' work rather than seeking the spotlight, and encouraging innovative ideas for improving health and health care in its home state. The Foundation's approach to grantmaking in New Jersey has significantly different emphases than its national approach. While in its national programs the Foundation issues Calls for Proposals that have the potential to shape policies, to build new fields, and to demonstrate innovative ideas that others might pick up, its approach in New Jersey is to respond to local initiatives and, to a great extent, to fund community-based programs. This approach offers a more receptive environment for a wide range of proposals, especially those that do not fall within the Foundation's national goals. This approach has both benefits and costs. These can be seen by examining four issues that arise from the Foundation's New Jersey grantmaking: What is an appropriate amount for a national foundation to give for programs in its own backyard? What are appropriate program priorities? What is an appropriate mechanism for making funding decisions? How visible should a national foundation be locally?

Funding Level

The first issue involves deciding how much of its funds a national foundation such as Robert Wood Johnson should devote to its own backyard. In 1990, the Foundation determined that, given past expenditures, a 3 percent level for out-of-program grants would be appropriate. Using historical spending patterns as a yardstick may be a rational way to determine current spending levels, but it has the potential drawback of freezing local grant-making at a level based only on history. However, the Foundation built in flexibility: the 3 percent is merely a target—a level that it should try to reach. Second, the 3 percent target applies only to out-of-program grants; in-program grants, including the New Jersey Health Initiatives, legacy grants, and, of course, grants to New Jersey applicants in national competitions are above and beyond the 3 percent. The exclusion of legacy grants in the 3 percent target is understandable, since the number of legacy grantees is finite, predetermined, and continuing, whereas the demand for out-of program grants to facilities and institutions is considerably less predictable. By excluding in-program grants from the 3 percent set-aside, these projects, in effect, compete for funds with the Foundation's national grantmaking portfolio.

Program Priorities

The second issue concerns the activities that fall within the guidelines for local grantmaking. The Foundation has program priorities in New Jersey different from those it has in other states. In New Jersey, the Foundation acts, for the most part, as a traditional community foundation, funding local charitable endeavors and using guidelines quite different from those it uses nationally. Its emphasis on charitable giving through the legacy and out-of-program mechanisms—whether or not they involve health—is markedly different from the Foundation's program priorities elsewhere. Even the New Jersey Health Initiatives, in which projects must fit within the Foundation's priorities, looks for community-based service activities and excludes grants for policy and research, which are a primary tool in many national programs.

Moreover, like community foundations that usually react to proposals that come over the transom, the Foundation makes grants that respond to requests coming from community organizations in New Jersey; this contrasts with its more structured and activist approach to national programs. Responding to the needs defined by local organizations is part of the definition of being a good corporate neighbor.

Some critics have commented that the approach the Foundation has adopted in New Jersey may deprive it of the opportunity to play a more decisive role in the state. In response to the challenge of making a greater impact in New Jersey, the Board approved an expanded scope for the New Jersey Health Initiatives in July 2001, adding three new elements: a community leadership program, capacity building for community organizations, and a strategic Call for Proposals in which each cycle will target a particular health or health care issue.

Mechanisms for Decision Making

A third issue is how to make decisions about what organizations and projects to fund. The Foundation's program staff is essentially removed from most New Jersey program development and decision making. Legacy and out-of-program grants do not go through the normal staff proposal review process; review and decisions are basically made by committees of the board of trustees. Decision making on New Jersey Health Initiatives grants is in the hands of an external program office, although members of the Foundation's program staff with relevant experience may be asked to comment on specific proposals.

The separation of the Foundation's program staff from grant-making in New Jersey has its pros and cons. It has the benefit of shielding the staff from involvement in projects that may have been submitted by friends or neighbors. In addition, the use of an expert advisory committee and a competitive review process for in-program grants funded under the New Jersey Health Initiatives maintains the credibility of the grantmaking process. However, the advantages brought by distancing the staff from local projects comes at a price: the Foundation loses the opportunity to apply its strategic and time-tested grantmaking process in New Jersey, and the staff is less able to share insights gained from its national programs with local audiences.

The Foundation's Visibility

Mark Murphy, executive director of the Fund for New Jersey, is not shy about expressing his admiration for the Robert Wood Johnson Foundation. However, he considers the Foundation's preference for remaining in the background among its less effective characteristics. He points out that the Foundation has learned much from projects all over the country that should inform the Foundation's potential to effect positive change in New Jersey. "The Robert Wood Johnson Foundation is uniquely positioned to provide expertise and resources to bring people together and make things happen," Murphy said. "The process that has protected the Foundation from the stickiness of engagement has also protected it from some of the potential achievements of engagement."

The Foundation's preference for low visibility is not unique to New Jersey. Indeed, it goes back to its first Board chairman, Gustav Lienhard, and was reaffirmed as recently as 1999 with the Board's adoption of a set of core values, including this: "We speak through our grantees and do not seek a high institutional profile." Without abandoning this core value, however, the Foundation could use the power of its New Jersey funding more strategically. Pauline Seitz, director of the New Jersey Health Initiatives through the end of 2000, took steps in this direction by using the Initiative's quasi-community foundation status to become active in the Council of New Jersey Grantmakers. As vice-president, she stimulated discussion about how New Jersey philanthropies could pool their assets for the good of the state.

How could the Foundation strengthen the impact of its New Jersey funding without losing the benefits of the approach that has evolved over the years? One way would be to adopt a strategic approach that would establish New Jersey as a discrete goal area, subject to the same incentives, constraints, and performance assessments that are applied to the national grantmaking processes. Two-way communications that would facilitate the sharing of experiences between New Jersey grantees and national program grantees could be built into the approach, and a budget process could be developed that would identify an appropriate level of resources needed to reach the goals.

A second approach would be to develop in selected localities in New Jersey what is referred to as a "place-based" type of grantmaking. Rather than taking one model and seeking to replicate it in many different sites, the place-based site approach takes many different types of interventions and implements them in a single place. The multiple interventions might yield synergies where the whole is greater than the sum of its parts. For several years, the Foundation has discussed applying this approach to children's health in a city in New Jersey. In July, 2001, the Board approved the Children's Futures program, which will focus exclusively on Trenton and bring to bear all that the Foundation has learned about improving the health of children between the ages of 0 and 3. This initiative might be risky because of the potential involvement of the Foundation in local affairs, but it could make a genuine and lasting contribution to the Foundation's home state.[3]

Notes

1. The source for material about the life of Robert Wood Johnson is Lawrence Foster, *Robert Wood Johnson: The Gentleman Rebel*. State College, PA: Lillian Press, 1999.
2. Ibid, p. 371.
3. The author would like to thank the following people for their insights and contributions toward this chapter: Len Fishman, Lawrence G. Foster, Ruby Hearn, Robert G. Hughes, Frank Karel, Terrance Keenan, Mark Murphy, Mary Quinn, Pauline Seitz, and Warren Wood.

Section Two

Programs

CHAPTER 9

Project ECHO: Bringing Specialists' Expertise to Underserved Rural Areas

Sara Solovitch

Editors' Introduction

One of the enduring problems of American medicine is how to provide care for people living in isolated, rural areas where medical resources are scarce. The problem is particularly acute for those with conditions requiring the skills of a specialist, most of whom tend to live in cities or near major medical centers. In many rural areas, if there is a doctor available at all, he or she is likely to be a general practitioner.

In this chapter, Sara Solovitch, a California-based journalist and freelance writer, tells the story of an innovative way of providing medical expertise in the treatment of complex illnesses suffered by people living in rural areas. Developed by Sanjeev Arora, a physician affiliated with the University of New Mexico School of Medicine and a leading expert on liver diseases, Project ECHO enables primary care physicians and nurses in rural New Mexico to consult, via videoconference, with specialists at the University of New Mexico Medical School about how best to treat their patients with hepatitis C. The project, whose scope has expanded to other diseases and other states, has been widely hailed as a breakthrough. Most recently, the Center for Medicare & Medicaid Innovation singled out Project ECHO for a Health Care Innovation Award, which comes with $8.5 million to enable further expansion of the project.

The partnership between Dr. Arora and the University of New Mexico School of Medicine is grounded in an extensive history of outreach to rural and low-income communities by the University of New Mexico. Its various initiatives include Vision 2020, a commitment to work with community partners to improve population health and health equity by 2020; a combined BA/MD program to encourage native New Mexicans to become physicians and to practice in rural and underserved areas; and a home visiting program for patients suffering from mental illness.

The Robert Wood Johnson Foundation has had a long interest in improving access to health care in rural areas, dating back to 1975 when it launched the Rural Practice Project to establish primary care practices in rural areas, and continuing through the mid-2000s with the Southern Rural Access Program that tested a range of approaches in a particularly difficult region. Over the past forty years, the Foundation has strengthened institutions, such as hospitals and nursing homes in rural areas; supported the development of health professionals such as nurse practitioners and community health aides who would serve in rural communities; provided incentives for physicians to practice in rural areas; and utilized distance learning via the Internet to train rural health professionals.

In the case of Project ECHO, the Foundation played a small but significant role. Project ECHO received its initial funding from the federal government's Agency for Healthcare Research and Quality and from the State of New Mexico. Through its pioneer team, which looks for groundbreaking ideas, the Foundation discovered the project and provided it with funds to expand beyond New Mexico and to address other diseases. The expansion is now under way, and the story is still unfolding.

Clustered at one end of a long Albuquerque conference table, a team of medical specialists from the University of
New Mexico gaze up at two 90-inch flat-screen TVs and welcome
a coterie of doctors, nurses, and physician assistants—all plugged
in from remote areas across the state, all waiting expectantly,
their patient files before them. Modeled on the idea of a "virtual
grand round," the specialists—a pharmacist, a psychiatrist, an
infectious disease specialist, and a nurse—sit flanked around Sanjeev Arora, a gastroenterologist and hepatologist (liver specialist)
and the force behind Project ECHO, a pioneering approach that
brings the expertise of an academic medical center to general
practitioners working in rural areas, coaching them to manage a
particularly difficult disease—hepatitis C.

One by one, the primary care providers present their cases.
Among them is Nii Tetteh Addy, a physician originally from
Ghana, now practicing in the backwater city of Carlsbad, near
the Texas border. Addy sits in his jam-packed office kitchenette,
squeezed up against a little table heaped with boxes of day-old
donuts and half-eaten bags of chips. It's been a long day. It is now
past five o'clock, and there are still patients waiting to see him.

When it is his turn, Addy turns off the mute button and
begins describing JD, a longtime heroin addict, who finally quit
only to discover that he has hepatitis C and cirrhosis of the
liver. The doctor continues on with the case of SS, a thirty-four-
year-old woman just diagnosed with hepatitis C. A few months
before, she managed to stop using meth. Now she's working on
quitting smoking. Addy recognizes that it is premature to seriously
consider treating either one of these patients for hepatitis C.

Earlier that day, he had checked in with Brad L., a patient he
had presented repeatedly to Project ECHO before finally obtaining approval to treat.[1] Brad was a handful, Addy acknowledged:
a fifty-seven-year-old with hepatitis C, Type 3 Genotype.[2] Brain
injury sustained as a combat veteran in Vietnam. Seizures as a

result of that head trauma. Impulsive. Unstable. Smoked two packs a day. Drank 18–24 beers a day. Occasional blackouts from drinking binges.

—ᨓ— The Case of Brad L.

Brad has no reluctance talking about his past or the fact that for a couple of decades he shot up a daily cocktail of cocaine and methamphetamine. But that, he insists, is not what gave him the hepatitis C—because he always knew better than to use a dirty needle. As a kid growing up in New Mexico, Brad got his First Aid certification by the time he was thirteen. During all those years that he shot meth, he made it his business to know exactly what he was injecting into his veins: usually a high-quality prescription pill obtained from one of the doctors he knew in Carlsbad.

Brad has long gray hair, a mouthful of missing teeth, and one eye that squints and looks a little bigger than the other. His body is covered with tattoos, most of them homemade blue, but here again he rejects the idea that this may have been how he got the disease. Instead, he points to his two-year stint in Vietnam, where, he says, "They used to line us up like cattle and give us the same hypodermic device for our vaccinations."

He gets riled up, squints rapidly, then catches himself, smiles self-deprecatingly, and forces himself to slow down. *Doesn't matter*. He got the diagnosis back in 2000, when he checked into rehab at a community-based outpatient clinic with the Department of Veterans Affairs in Colorado Springs. Even then, Brad knew what it signified. His mother had died of the same disease some years back. Now, facing the same risk, he wasn't so sure he wanted the treatment.

Not that it would be so easy to come by in his neck of the woods. Carlsbad is an isolated town in the southeast corner of New Mexico, better known as a geological nuclear-waste site than as a nucleus for high-end medical care. Thirty-two of the state's thirty-three counties are officially listed as Medically Underserved

Areas by the federal Health Resources and Services Administration, and Eddy County, of which Carlsbad is the seat, is one.[3]

As a state, New Mexico is one of the poorest in the nation. It also happens to have one of the nation's highest rates of hepatitis C, a viral disease that leads to inflammation of the liver. In its early stages, most people don't even know they have it. The virus can fester in the liver for up to a couple of decades, doing its damage while giving few, if any, symptoms. Left untreated, it can lead to cirrhosis of the liver, liver cancer, and liver failure. In the United States, 3.2 million people have hepatitis C. Thirty-two thousand of them live in New Mexico, but fewer than 5 percent receive treatment.

> More people in America die from hepatitis C than from AIDS—in 2007, for example, there were more than 15,000 hepatitis C deaths, higher than previous estimates and surpassing the nearly 13,000 AIDS deaths. Hepatitis C is a silent disease in the early years. The Centers for Disease Control and Prevention is considering recommending that all Americans born between 1945 and 1965 get a one-time blood test to check if their livers harbor the virus.

In medical sociology parlance, hepatitis C is what is known as a shame-based disease. Many of the people who have it are America's untouchables. Transmitted through the blood of an infected person (often by way of shared needles), the disease frequently infects drug addicts, sex workers, the homeless, and the incarcerated. Primary care providers generally refrain from treating hepatitis C, regarding it as a disease that requires a specialist's expertise—largely because the treatment regimen is so complex and grueling.

The main drug, interferon—a protein that boosts the immune system—is associated with a host of physical, psychiatric, and neurological side effects, including depression and thoughts of suicide. Substance abuse, smoking, and mental-health issues are common problems among hepatitis C patients, and each one needs to be addressed before treatment can begin. In Brad's case, he had to be weaned off alcohol, regularly attending Twelve Step meetings and getting six months' sobriety under his belt. He had to quit smoking (tobacco depletes red blood cells and lowers the body's oxygen levels), undergo psychiatric testing, and agree to take antidepressants. "For a long time, he resisted all these things," Addy tells his listeners. "But it got to the point where he realized we wouldn't treat him unless he got help."

By the time Brad got around to seeking treatment, there weren't many choices. Carlsbad had only one gastroenterologist, and as far as anybody knew, he didn't treat hepatitis. He left town in 2004, the same year Addy arrived as an employee of Presbyterian Medical Services—a nonprofit organization of primary care clinics throughout New Mexico. Addy had left Ghana to attend medical school at New York College of Osteopathic Medicine, and then trained at Bay Regional Medical Center in Bay City, Michigan. Of the ten or so newly minted primary care physicians who arrived in Carlsbad that year, he says he is the only one who remains. A little formal, he carries himself in an erect posture and speaks softly, in a heavy but understandable West African accent. After four years, he has managed to buck the prevailing winds and open his own clinic, a nondescript building sandwiched between two auto supply stores, where he sees patients twelve hours a day, five days a week. His colleagues around the state quietly wonder how he manages to pay his nurse and office staff and still make a living, because Addy is known far and wide for never turning anyone away.

He still remembers his first day on the job at Presbyterian, when, going through charts, he discovered he had been assigned eight patients with hepatitis C. "One after the other," he says, still awed at the number. "I said to myself, 'How could this be?'" I didn't think you would see this unless you went to a hepatitis C clinic.

"Continuity of care was lacking," Addy continues. "Providers came and went. It was overwhelming. I began to keep track of my hepatitis C cases and in three months I had about 120 patients. I went to the health department to inquire about prevalence. They said yes, it was very prevalent, but nothing was being done about it. There didn't seem to be any interest."

After a couple false starts, he found his way to Project ECHO, a new program based out of the University of New Mexico in Albuquerque. It was the brainchild of another transplanted doctor, Sanjeev Arora, who, like Addy, had been jolted by the sheer number of hepatitis C patients he was seeing—and turning away.

—⚘— The Development of Project ECHO

"There was an eight-month wait to see me," says Arora, a professor and former executive vice chairman of the department of internal medicine at the University of New Mexico School of Medicine and one of the world's experts in hepatitis C. "People would have to drive 250 miles each way, and if it was genotype 1, they'd have to make eighteen trips . . . I treated as many as I could. But people were basically dying from lack of expertise."

In 2004, Arora launched a program to treat those patients in an entirely different way. Dubbed Project ECHO (Extension for Community Healthcare Outcomes), it has evolved within just a few years into an innovative model for transforming a deeply troubled health care system. It has been adopted by major academic medical centers around the country and been embraced by the Veterans Health Administration for a variety of diseases, including diabetes, asthma, and chronic-pain management.

At age fifty-five, Arora is a private, reserved man who rarely raises his voice. But when the subject turns to Project ECHO—as it inevitably does—he is passionate and charismatic. As one of fifty-four gastroenterologists (and only three hepatologists) in New Mexico, Arora was frustrated by the fact that he could see just a fraction of the hepatitis C patients referred to him. There had to be a better way, he thought—a way to make himself a "force multiplier," as he puts it, employing a military term describing a factor that significantly increases the effectiveness of a combat unit.

But it wasn't until 2003, when his younger daughter went off to college, that he found the time to tackle a long-term solution. As Arora describes it, he and his wife, Madhu Arora, an internal medicine physician, went away on a weekend retreat. During that brief getaway, Arora found himself reflecting on the issues most important to him—and how he wanted to spend the rest of his life. "Was there a way I could amplify my own expertise so that my decades of experience could be applied to many more people?" he wondered. "My goal was to serve every person in New Mexico with hepatitis C. And I thought, my god, if I could do that I would have a model to serve complex diseases around the world!"

By the end of the weekend, he had his answer. Though he didn't have a name for it yet, it was in every important way the prototype for Project ECHO—a "knowledge network" in which primary care doctors, nurses, physician assistants, and nurse practitioners from around the state could join in on a weekly videoconference with a team of hepatitis C experts from the University of New Mexico. Arora saw it as a means of sharing best practices within a larger community of providers, modeled on the close supervision that young doctors routinely get in medical school and residency programs.

"You cannot make gastroenterologists with lectures," he explains. "But if a mentor holds your hand, that process is extraordinarily facilitated. So I said, why should we not bring case-based learning back into the lives of the rural provider by comanaging patients with them?"

For the next couple of years, Arora logged thousands of miles, visiting the four corners of New Mexico from its mountains and buttes in the north to the gray desert in the south. Every two weeks, he got in his car, a 1993 Lexus, and drove. He visited hospitals where he talked to CEOs and offered free grand rounds in gastroenterology. He called upon primary care providers in their offices, often waiting for them to finish with their patients so they could join him at a local restaurant, where he would continue his pitch with a portable projector in tow. Once he got a commitment from providers, he followed up with calls to their bosses to open up a couple hours a week in their schedule when they could be freed from seeing patients. "I would say, 'Let's find a day that causes the least disruption for you.' I fitted my schedule around theirs."

In this dogged, implacable way, he attracted a core of passionate idealists, physicians who, like himself, were committed to bringing health care to the poor and underserved. In fact, some of those doctors had come to New Mexico for exactly that purpose. Arora certainly had. Prior to moving to Albuquerque in 1993, he had been a staff physician at New England Medical Center and an associate professor at Tufts University School of Medicine. "I knew that if I left Boston not many patients would suffer," he says, shrugging. "I came to New Mexico because I was told that 20 percent of the people here have no health insurance."

That idealism was planted in childhood, when Arora accompanied his physician father, Ramrakha, a leader in the Indian government's eradication of smallpox, in his travels to remote towns and villages throughout the entire subcontinent. As a child himself, young Sanjeev witnessed the sight of children who were dehydrated and dying from cholera. The poverty and social disparities horrified him, and he knew he would commit his life to making a difference.

His mother, Sudarshan Arora, served as an additional role model. A retired obstetrician/gynecologist, she owns a private maternity hospital in Delhi, where it's her custom to treat poor patients free of charge—while billing the wealthy ones a hefty fee. In 1947, the fifteen-year-old Sudarshan had fled the newly created state of Pakistan and arrived in Delhi with her family. Her school records had been left behind in the rush and she had no papers to document her education. Determined to go to medical school, she took matters into her own hands. She tracked down the residence of Prime Minister Jawaharlal Nehru, and when Nehru emerged from the house and got into his chauffeur-driven Hindustan Ambassador, the teenage girl stepped in front of it and refused to move until he opened the car window and heard her out. He signed her school admission papers on the spot, and she began her premedical studies.

Smiling a little self-consciously, Arora acknowledges that he probably inherited his mother's self-confidence. "People believe that the walls of the system are impenetrable and that you have to live within them," he says. "I don't believe that. I believe in tinkering with the knowledge monopoly."

—⌇— Project ECHO and the Treatment of Hepatitis C in New Mexico

Arora launched Project ECHO with $1.5 million in funding from the federal Agency for Healthcare Research and Quality (AHRQ) in 2004.[4] With this grant, he recruited a group of specialists: a pharmacist, a psychiatrist, an infectious-disease expert, and an information technology consultant. The core of the project is the weekly videoconference linking primary care providers in the countryside with specialists at the University of New Mexico. In addition, Project ECHO holds a biweekly orientation meeting that is intended to spread the word, drum up interest, and tutor potential converts.

In these biweekly meetings, Arora draws freely from theories garnered from the business and academic worlds, holding forth on such ideas as "the Pareto Principle" (also known as the 80–20 rule or law of the vital few); "adult learning theory" (upon which Project ECHO is based); the "self-efficacy theory" (advanced by Stanford University psychologist Albert Bandura); and "the zone of proximal development," a concept—attributed to Soviet psychologist Lev Vygotsky—which states that a child follows an adult's example until it develops the ability to do certain tasks without help.

Arora, who holds a master's degree in management science from Tulane University, has obviously assimilated the concepts that tie these principles together in a meaningful way. But when young doctors attend Project ECHO's orientation meetings, their typical response isn't so much "But of course, this bears out Vygotsky's theories of how a young surgeon learns her craft"; it's more like, "Well, duh, this is social networking as applied to medicine."

"Chronic disease management is a team sport, more like soccer than golf," says Arora, turning, as he often does, to metaphor. "The data demands collaboration. Something magic happens when you bring a nurse, psychiatrist, and doctor together." He pauses a thoughtful moment. "It's like if you eat sugar and then flour. It doesn't make cake."

Sometimes, to the surprise of even those directly involved in the process, the most difficult patients—people like Brad L., who for decades struggled with substance abuse, high-stress relationships, and personal demons—eventually come around. An outside observer may well question how it happens, but the answer is obvious to those who watch from the sidelines, week after week. "Good solid advice," asserts Davin Quinn, a psychiatrist and psychosomatic medicine specialist with Project ECHO. "It's someone planting the idea that you can change. It sounds ridiculously simple, but that's what they teach you in medical school. If you just tell the patient repeatedly, it sinks in."

At its core, too, the idea of Project ECHO, like all good ideas, is simple and elegant—an almost organic use of available technology. Arora is interested in nothing less than worldwide replication: if he teaches ten centers how to do a Project ECHO, and each of them teaches ten more centers, before long there are a hundred new Project ECHOs. And, that, he says, is how you change the world.

But first, Arora had to bring about change in New Mexico. That is now well under way. Partnerships have quickly developed between the University of New Mexico and the state's prisons, its health department, the Indian Health Service, and numerous primary care providers. By 2012, there were 250 clinicians throughout New Mexico logging in on a weekly basis to the Project ECHO videoconferencing line, using a secure, Internet-based audiovisual network. And it was happening in places in the state as distant geographically and sociologically as the outskirts of Albuquerque, Carlsbad, and Española.

South Valley

First Choice Community Heathcare lies just a few miles from the University of New Mexico, in South Valley, but it seems more like country than city. Dr. Vanessa Jacobsohn eats lunch, a cold bagel and cream cheese, at her desk. A rooster crows in the distance. Jacobsohn, a soft-spoken woman of thirty-five, her dark hair pulled back in a ponytail, is waiting for a call from an insurance company that she hopes will give her authorization to treat a hepatitis C patient already approved by Project ECHO. But the company has been holding up treatment for days, insisting that the treating physician be either a gastroenterologist or a hepatitis C specialist.

A family medicine doctor just four years out of residency, Jacobsohn still remembers one of her first hepatitis C cases: a sixty-year-old Hispanic man who had been infected with the virus for decades and was well along in cirrhosis. His family convinced him to disregard doctors' advice—better, they told him, to go back to Mexico. And so he did, opting for an alternative therapy involving some kind of shock treatment. By the time he returned to his young doctor in Albuquerque, his virus load had significantly increased.

"We convinced him to begin treatment," Jacobsohn says. "I was really nervous because we convinced this man to put his trust in us." The man's trust was well earned. Six months after treatment, he was free of the virus.

These days, about half of Jacobsohn's caseload involves hepatitis C, but she still occasionally catches the raised eyebrows among older specialists, including her uncle, a California gastroenterologist. "Really, interferon?" Granted, it is not an easy medication to control. Things can go bad fast. But oversight from Project ECHO is so consistent that Jacobsohn says she's never felt like she was working without a safety net. "From the beginning, they made it so clear about how the protocol works. And they are so cautious. I honestly never felt afraid, like it was a big risk. There is always a pharmacist, a psychiatrist, and a hepatologist guiding you, backing up the major decisions."

And unlike the intimidation she felt in medical school—the fear that by speaking up and asking a stupid question she might be ridiculed and shot down—Jacobsohn marvels at the nurturing environment she has met online. "Not long after I started with Project ECHO, I realized it wasn't going to be like that. These physicians are world renowned and brilliant, but they never make you feel stupid for asking a question."

It is not easy to create a warm and supportive videoconference atmosphere, but Project ECHO has made it its business to do just that. Before speaking, the participating specialists are encouraged to pause, count to five seconds, enough time to allow the presenters to unmute their phones and ask their questions.

"It is very frightening to present to people in a remote place," notes Quinn. "You're afraid that someone is listening to and assessing your clinical presentation. There's a fear of judgment and inadequacy, of falling on one's face and everyone hearing it. Plus, you don't have the nonverbal cues you get when you're in a room full of people."

But though Arora is a world expert on hepatitis, he never speaks down to the providers who tune in each week. Instead, says Quinn, he addresses them in a clear and concise way, explaining what's happening to their patients as they go through treatment. "He's extremely compelling," says Quinn.

Española

Just shy of ninety miles to the northeast of Albuquerque is Española, where physician assistant Debra Newman also serves as part of the ECHO team. Española lies in Georgia O'Keeffe country, but it's equally famous, at least within New Mexico, as the heroin capital of the United States. Doctors and nurses describe a town where opiate use is the cultural norm, where some families set aside an "injection room" the way other families have a music room, and where it's not unheard of for grandmothers to teach their fifteen-year-old granddaughters how to tie off their arms and shoot up. Rio Arriba County has long held the highest ranking of drug overdose fatalities in the nation: 51.1 per 100,000, compared with a national average of 7.3.

The Rio Arriba Health Clinic, on the edge of town, is surrounded by a seven-foot wire fence topped with barbed wire; signs posted throughout the lobby and examination rooms declare that "Narcotic drugs are not stocked at this facility." For the past four years, Newman has been making the twenty-mile weekly commute from Santa Fe to the clinic, where her caseload has consisted mostly of substance abuse and hepatitis C patients. She says she could easily see twenty-five patients a week instead of the two permitted for time's sake. In January 2012, she had twelve hepatitis C patients on interferon and ribavirin (an antiviral drug that prevents the virus from replicating itself), and saw many more on an almost daily basis. "Half the patients know they have it, the other half don't know," she says. "And the half who know they have it don't want treatment. I hear things like, 'My neighbor had it and it's terrible. It's going to kill me, it's going to make me sick.'"

"Our strategy is this," Newman said. "We have a great captive audience because we have a huge problem with addiction and a lot of people who want to get on Suboxone. The minute they ask, we test them for hepatitis." Suboxone, a form of buprenorphine, approved in 2002 as an opiate replacement, is widely preferred to methadone, which must be given in a clinic setting and is itself an addictive, sedating drug. Suboxone can be prescribed by primary care physicians and taken at home; the potential for overdose is nonexistent, and it is nonsedating.

On a recent Monday morning, almost all of Newman's patients have or suspect they have hepatitis. Carlos T., a fifty-nine-year-old man with advanced cirrhosis of the liver, is waiting stoically. He has proved a difficult patient, though he seems inordinately pleasant and happy to see Newman. Months earlier, before beginning treatment, he assured her that—as required—he had seen a dentist in Mexico and been given a clean bill of oral health. He hadn't. Now, all his teeth were falling out. He had also ignored the doctors' advice to consume a high-fat diet for the first twelve weeks of treatment; the protease inhibitor he was taking required such a diet to enhance its absorption. A dietician had been called in to work with him. She had recommended a daily snack of guacamole and chips, but Carlos had opted instead for an afternoon banana.

As a result, four weeks after treatment he still had signs of the virus in his bloodstream, while others on the same regimen were free of it. Newman was disturbed to see that his blood pressure had shot up and his potassium had plunged. Carlos's wife had called to report that he was depressed and rarely left the house. After a few minutes, Newman discovered that he was taking only two ribavirin tablets each morning. "No, you have to take three or you won't clear the virus in your body," she tells him, before phoning his grown daughter, who translated to make sure he understood.

Then Newman gave Carlos a short questionnaire, the CES-D, a self-reporting survey for measuring depressive symptoms. While he checked the questions off in Spanish, she moved next door, where a thirty-two-year-old named Ricardo was waiting to see her for the first time. He was a large, imposing man with several homemade tattoos, including two prominent ones: on his right hand, "13 SUR"—Southern United Raza, the Surenos gang; and under his right eye, a little blue tear.

The tear, he explained, was in commemoration of his grand-father, who had died of hepatitis C while Ricardo was doing time in a juvenile facility twelve years before. Ricardo volunteered that the tear was also symbolic of having killed someone. In prison, he explained, tattoos were kind of like a suit and tie on Wall Street; you needed them to hold your own. Now that he was out, he was considering having it removed. "It's hard to get a job if people think I killed someone," he said.

He ran through his history in unapologetic fashion, admitting that yes, he used to inject cocaine and methamphetamine—but he stopped at least seven years ago. He was diagnosed with hep-atitis C in 2001 and didn't think too much about it. But then, just seven months ago, he had flu symptoms and went to the local emergency room where a standard blood test reconfirmed the orig-inal diagnosis. Ricardo was a different person now—a Christian rapper at his church; a family man with a one-year-old daughter ("the light of my life") and a girlfriend, who also had hepatitis C. "We've been together two years. We heard it was curable," he said.

"Up to six months ago, genotype 1 was the hardest to treat," Newman said, "but there are new medications available and it's curable 75 percent of the time. But you have to be really on top of it. I don't know if *I* could do it, to be honest," she added, looking him square in the eye. "You have to be very organized. You have to take the medications every eight hours for twelve weeks, and if you miss a few doses you're done with the treatment."

Ricardo met her gaze. "I am definitely committed to the program. You don't have to worry about that."

His BMI was 32, a little high for the treatment. He would need to drop at least fifteen pounds. Not a problem, he said. Smoking? Maybe a puff a week. What about alcohol? Never touched the stuff. Depression? "I'm the kind of person who cheers others up."

Newman ordered a battery of tests but she was clearly impressed by the way he presented himself. He appeared a strong candidate for treatment and she imagined that she would be presenting his case at the next Project ECHO clinic. She shook his hand as she left the room, but halfway down the hall, she was suddenly struck with a realization: she knew the girlfriend.

"It's Leslie! She came in with her mother and tested positive for benzodiazepine—which she flatly denied. She has significant psychological issues and needs to lose at least seventy pounds before we can treat her." Back in her office, Newman pulled out her files and saw that Leslie had recently visited the local ER following a physical "altercation" with her boyfriend. Ricardo's case was suddenly looking more complicated.

—⌇— Beyond Hepatitis C and New Mexico

As the idea took off and word about this new program grew, Project ECHO began holding biweekly orientation meetings. A recent one was attended by a disparate group of visitors, including an anesthesiologist and a family practice physician (both assigned to the U.S. Army in Fort Campbell, Kentucky); a chronic pain nurse from Cleveland, Virginia; the president of the World Gastroenterology Organization (who traveled from Uruguay to learn about the program); two high-level executives from Molina Healthcare, a California-based national insurance company that works with low-income families and individuals; a grant writer; and a technology engineer.

The model has spread to other academic centers, including the University of Washington, the University of Chicago, the University of Utah, Harvard University, and the University of Nevada. Eleven regions of the Veterans Administration— including Cleveland, Ohio; New Haven, Connecticut; and Ann Arbor, Michigan—have adopted Project ECHO, and medical emissaries have come to Albuquerque from India and Uruguay. Arora is also in discussions with medical leaders in Brazil and Ireland.

Meanwhile, Project ECHO has expanded beyond hepatitis C and now covers additional diseases, including asthma, mental illness, chronic pain, diabetes, cardiovascular risk reduction, high-risk pregnancy, HIV/AIDS, pediatric obesity, autism, rheumatology, and substance abuse. The VA uses the model to treat chronic pain, diabetes, hepatitis C, and heart failure.

Arora's staff clearly holds him in high regard. "As a gastroenterologist, Sanjeev could walk out of here and make half a million a year giving colonoscopies to fifty-year-old men," declares John Brown, the project's operations director. "Most people like him are working their way up to the National Institutes of Health. He's taken a huge risk in his career. He was executive vice chair of internal medicine. The next step was chancellorship. He threw all that away to get involved with Project ECHO."

In fact, it was a risk that has paid off handsomely. In 2009, the Ashoka Foundation, an international association of social entrepreneurs, named Arora an honorary fellow and credited Project ECHO as a disruptive innovation that is changing the way health care is delivered. The Robert Wood Johnson Foundation followed shortly after, awarding Project ECHO a $5 million grant to replicate the ECHO model in academic medical centers outside of New Mexico, beginning with the University of Washington Medical School—and also to expand its work to include asthma, diabetes, chronic pain and headache, high-risk pregnancy, integrated addictions, psychiatry, and rheumatology.

The Foundation urged Project ECHO leaders to take those clinics to "industrial strength" throughout New Mexico. "At the heart of this," says Risa Lavizzo-Mourey, president and CEO of the Robert Wood Johnson Foundation, "is a team approach to delivering care, one that depends on a lot of different providers bringing their expertise to the case of very complex, chronically ill patients."

Adds Nancy Barrand, who, as special adviser for program development, oversees Project ECHO at the Foundation: "It is significant that Dr. Arora started with hepatitis C, working with patients whom no one else treated or wanted to treat. He started in a part of the market that no one else was paying attention to, and built a model that worked. And because it worked so well, it just naturally started to infuse into the rest of the system and we have what we have today."

⟿ The Significance of Project ECHO

Project ECHO has grown from an organization of five people in 2004 to a staff of more than seventy in 2012. With that kind of growth, there have been some growing pains. But throughout, Arora has freely bestowed the ECHO logo and method to any organization that wants to use it. "As long as you want to monopolize knowledge, it has little impact," he says. "We have to be willing to break the monopoly of knowledge that exists. Breaking that monopoly and sharing it freely for public benefit, without necessarily charging anybody for it, doing it at low cost on public dollars, would be much more cost effective."

He is arguing, he says, for a new kind of health care system—one that will reconfigure the role of the primary care doctor in America. Arora wants to create a network of primary care doctors, each with a subspecialty or interest in rheumatology, chronic pain, or hepatitis C, who will build relationships with academic centers. "We think primary care is an embattled specialty," says Arora. "But you cannot encourage a system where all are specialists." In this vision of a new health care order, there is a lot of room, too, for nurse practitioners and physician assistants.

"He's changed the rules of the game," says the Foundation's Barrand. Though traditional telemedicine was once touted as a game changer, it failed to change the actual delivery of health care. Indeed, says Barrand, telemedicine is a "limiting technology" that locked health care delivery in place. As typically practiced, she says, telemedicine allows a physician to see patients only on a one-to-one basis, thus restricting the number they can treat. Project ECHO, in contrast, changes the entire paradigm, allowing a specialist to consult on up to a dozen or more complicated cases in a couple of hours—while leaving the primary care provider in control of his or her own patient.

Barrand credits Arora's skill in team building as one of the main reasons for Project ECHO's success. "We have too many specialists and too few primary care doctors, and this is one of the better ways—if not the only way—we'll be able to expand capacity and improve quality of care at the same time. He does a lot of work with the paraprofessionals to make the primary care physicians more effective. It's why he's able to change the organization of care. It's how he passes knowledge all the way down the chain."

The model's effectiveness was demonstrated in a prospective cohort study, published in the *New England Journal of Medicine* in June 2011, which reported that patients treated under Project ECHO had similar and even slightly better outcomes than patients treated at an academic medical center. According to that article, 58.2 percent of the 261 patients treated at rural sites showed a sustained viral response (a complete and permanent cure), as compared with 57.5 percent of those treated at the University of New Mexico's hepatitis C clinic.[5]

Coda

In early 2012, with the guidance of Project ECHO specialists, Dr. Addy was able to instruct Brad L. in how to inject himself in the stomach once a week with interferon and ribavirin. "Today's my third injection and by tonight I will be hurting like total hell," Brad says, almost cheerfully. "Every part of my body will hurt. My bones will ache, my nose will run, my throat'll be dry. It usually lasts three days." But within four weeks, his system was free of the virus. His treatment would continue another six months before he could be declared cured.

And after four years of working in Española's Rio Arriba Clinic, physician assistant Debra Newman decided she had had enough. Lacking the administrative or nursing support she felt she needed to do her job, in early 2012 she gave notice and began packing up. She would continue to work with Project ECHO in Santa Fe, where she had accepted a hospital job managing chronic pain.

Even so, in her voice there was the slight sound of regret. "You never quite know what's going to happen one day to the next," Newman said on her second to last day at the clinic. "I had a woman in today who'd been on Suboxone. She was the hero of Suboxone therapy—she weaned herself off Suboxone, started eight Narcotics Anonymous groups in this town, and was going to school to become a therapist. A lovely, lovely person!"

"She came in today for what I thought was going to be her first hepatitis C visit. And as soon as I walked into the room, she fell into my arms sobbing. Her back had been hurting and someone gave her a Percocet. Now she's back on opiates, as bad as ever. I held her and told her, this just isn't your time."

Later that day, Newman sat at her desk, under a Happy Hanukkah banner, and made her final call-in to Project ECHO's hepatitis C clinic. She related what had just happened, said her good-byes, thanked everyone for their help, and promised to stay in touch.

Three hundred miles away, in his crowded Carlsbad office kitchenette, Nii Tetteh Addy pushed himself away from his little table, faced the webcam mounted on the wall, and saluted her.

Notes

1. In the interest of confidentiality, names and initials of patients have been changed.
2. There are three main kinds of hepatitis in the United States: Hepatitis A, B, and C. Hepatitis C is actually the name given to a range of similar viruses, categorized by genotypes 1, 2, and 3. Genotype 1 is by far the most common.
3. Every county except Los Alamos has at least one medically underserved area in it, but not all of every county is designated as medically underserved.

4. The federal grant required a match, which was met by a three-year $900,000 grant from the New Mexico Legislature and a three-year $600,000 commitment of in-kind services from the University of New Mexico School of Medicine. In 2006, the New Mexico Legislature agreed to provide recurring funding—now at $900,000 per year—for Project ECHO. AHRQ provided another $1.5 million in 2007 and again in 2008. In 2012, Project ECHO won a Health Care Innovation Award from the Center for Medicare & Medicaid Innovation; it comes with $8.5 million over a three-year period.

5. Arora, S., and others. "Outcomes of treatment for Hepatitis C virus infection by primary care providers." *New England Journal of Medicine*, 2011, *364*, 2199–2206.

CHAPTER 10

The Food Trust: Increasing the Availability of Healthy Food

Will Bunch

Editors' Introduction

Even to those familiar with the situation, the extent and health consequences of obesity in the United States are shocking. More than one out of every three adults in this country is obese, up from one in ten fifty years ago. One in six children is obese, up from one in twenty only thirty years ago. Obesity-related illnesses, particularly diabetes, have risen dramatically, straining the health care system and causing untold personal tragedies to families. Equally important, obesity has become a byproduct of economic and racial disparities: it is far more prevalent in poor communities and among minorities.

Much of the problem, it is clear, has to do with the environment in which people, especially low-income people, live. If playgrounds or streets are dangerous, or after-school programs are not available, children will stay indoors and watch TV. If fresh fruits and vegetables are not easily available, families won't buy them. Hence, many of the obesity-reduction interventions favored by government and philanthropy focus on changing the environment so that healthier foods become more accessible and physical activity more easily available.[1]

One of the more promising approaches is bringing supermarkets to poor, inner-cities neighborhoods whose residents have little access to the kinds of healthy foods that supermarkets can easily stock. The Food Trust, which started more than twenty years ago, has been a pioneer in developing the approach in Pennsylvania. Based on The Food Trust's apparent success in bringing supermarkets and other healthy food outlets to underserved areas, the Robert Wood Johnson Foundation awarded several million dollars, beginning in 2006, to expand its activities to eight additional states.

The process may sound simple, but in practice, it is a very difficult one that involves zoning codes, complex financing transactions, and local politics, among other elements. Perhaps most important, it involves developing partnerships between government agencies and the private sector, something that is relatively new for the Robert Wood Johnson Foundation. In the past, the Foundation has worked extensively with government, but it has little experience collaborating with business and has been proceeding cautiously. Its work with The Food Trust is giving the Foundation experience in collaborating with a new, and in today's world, increasingly important partner.

In this chapter, Will Bunch, a journalist with the *Philadelphia Daily News* and most recently the author of *October 1, 2011: The Battle of the Brooklyn Bridge*, tells the story of The Food Trust from its beginning in Philadelphia's Reading Market to the present day. In addition to telling the story of The Food Trust, Bunch examines one of the current controversies in the field—whether inner cities really are "food deserts" whose residents are deprived of healthy food choices—and how it affects the need for supermarkets in inner cities.

Note

1. See Isaacs, S. L. and Swartz, A. C. "On the Front Lines of Childhood Obesity." *American Journal of Public Health*, 2010, *100*, 2018.

In 1992, Duane Perry, a thirty-seven-year-old graduate of Penn State with a master's degree in city planning from Harvard University and a track record of working with nonprofits, had just won a battle to save Philadelphia's landmark Reading Terminal Market, the century-old market located beneath what was once an iconic central rail terminal. Its rows of stalls selling farm-fresh produce, butchered meats, and the day's catch filled Center City with a rich aroma that was considered as much a part of Philadelphia's fabric as the Liberty Bell or cheesesteaks. As head of the market's merchants' trade association, Perry wanted to pay the city back for its support of his efforts to keep the market open as the new Pennsylvania Convention Center renovated the train shed overhead. And he had a lot of energy to channel into a new cause.

"I thought it would be great if the market did more," recalls Perry. Around that time he read a series of articles in the *Wall Street Journal* about urban neighborhoods that were without supermarkets—and the kinds of fresh foods readily available in the Reading Terminal Market. So he established the Reading Terminal Farmers' Market Trust as a kind of a win-win—creating new customers for the market's vendors and also providing a valuable public service to the urban poor. "Many of the vendors I worked with were passionate about providing food to people, so this resonated with them," he says. The initial farmers' market created by Perry's venture was at the Tasker Homes, a crime-ridden public housing project southwest of Center City.

Over the next decade, Perry expanded the one-day-a-week farmers' market to half a dozen locations, but customers made it clear they really wanted the everyday convenience and selection of a full-service supermarket in their neighborhood. "What we were hearing from people," says Yael Lehmann, the current executive director of The Food Trust who has worked for the nonprofit since 2001, "was, 'Well, it's great that you're here for one day a week for four hours, but this isn't really cutting it.'" By the early 2000s, Perry's effort had been rebranded as The Food Trust to reflect a broader mission that included opening new food outlets, especially supermarkets—as both a source of nutrition and also as a driver of job creation in poor neighborhoods.

—⁓— The Food Trust Develops in Pennsylvania

By the dawn of the new millennium it was clear that the lack of urban grocery options—a trend that had begun in the 1960s and 1970s—had passed a point of no return; one 1998 study revealed that urban neighborhoods now had about 55 percent of the supermarket square footage found in the suburbs,[1] and the Department of Agriculture says that today 23.5 million Americans do not have a supermarket within a mile of their home.[2]

Experts had no simple explanation for why this happened. Rather, the death of the urban supermarket seemed to be the result of a perfect storm of negative factors: higher costs for security and job training, inability to sell more lucrative luxury goods, consolidations and bankruptcies in the food industry, and a push for more profitable superstores of forty-five thousand square feet or more, or close to double the typical city supermarket footprint. In an industry that typically thrives on high volume and a low profit margin (just 1 or 2 percent), these negative factors led to a downward spiral in which supermarkets fell into grime-coated disrepair and then shut down altogether.

"For a long time, population declines and the general neglect of urban areas made things harder," says Jeff Brown, the CEO of Brown's Super Stores, which operates ShopRite markets through-out the Philadelphia region. "And because the picture looked bleak, nobody invested in the stores." In 2002, The Food Trust and the United Way invited Brown and other Philadelphia-area supermarket executives to join a Food Marketing Task Force on how to bring stores back to these "food deserts," as places without access to healthy, affordable food have come to be known.

Brown—a fourth-generation grocer whose family then owned four suburban stores—recalls being shocked at the cynicism expressed by some of the other attendees. "Look, we know this can't work," he recalls an executive from a major local chain whispering to him before the first meeting. "Just smile and nod your head."

Instead, the meeting inspired Brown. Calling the defeatism about the urban food system "practically un-American," he was moved to take a closer look at a problem he hadn't given much thought to before that day. First, he paid a visit to a poverty-stricken stretch of Southwest Philadelphia, which is in the flight path of the city's airport, where the particularly cynical executive's chain ran an underperforming grocery that was about to close. Despite discouraging reports about gun crime in the parking lot and widespread community distrust, Brown was determined to buy the location and come up with creative answers to its long-standing problems.

He convinced about two hundred residents to attend a community meeting. The meeting was quite heated at times. But the white supermarket CEO won over his predominantly African American future customers by promising to address their concerns—for example, cutting back the rarely used deli and greatly expanding fish offerings. "They had a Starbucks and a sushi bar," Brown says. "It made no sense." His idea for the crime problem was completely outside the box; his Southwest Philadelphia ShopRite would sponsor a gun buyback. The first one took about four to five hundred firearms off the streets; then, as Brown expanded his Philadelphia locations, the running total grew exponentially—and his stores have been largely free of serious crime.

Brown had a laundry list of other ideas—stricter gun laws and improved mass transit, for example—but when he presented the list to State Representative Dwight Evans, an influential Philadelphia lawmaker and advocate for urban development, Evans chuckled. "Governments aren't good at fixing things," he told Brown. "What we are good at is putting money aside."

Such discussions fed into the work of the Food Marketing Task Force that Brown served on with forty other key stakeholders. The task force recommended a statewide initiative to fund fresh food retail development. Evans championed the recommendation. The result was a successful legislative push for something that had never been tried elsewhere in the United States: the Pennsylvania Fresh Food Financing Initiative, a $120-million public-private partnership. Its innovative formula included $30 million in seed money from the Pennsylvania Department of Community & Economic Development and $90 million through The Reinvestment Fund, which comprised funding from banks including JPMorgan Chase, PNC, and Wachovia; the federal New Market Tax Credit Program; and a variety of other public and private sources. The Food Trust played, and continues to play, a critical role in administering the program by soliciting grocers and other key players to get involved and then prescreening applications to ensure they go to the areas of greatest need.

Authorized by the Pennsylvania legislature in 2004, the Fresh Food Financing Initiative provides grants of up to $250,000 and low-interest loans ranging in size from $25,000 to $7.5 million to reduce start-up costs for supermarket projects and other healthy food outlets in underserved locales across the state—not just in urban areas such as Philadelphia but also in the depressed former steel towns of western Pennsylvania and the remote rural areas in between. The projects selected receive grants and loans that can be used for feasibility or market studies; land assembly, acquisition, and other predevelopment costs; equipment and construction; and start-up expenses such as employee recruitment and training. ShopRite's Brown, who now travels widely to advise community leaders and supermarket entrepreneurs, said the seed money to reduce start-up costs is often the difference between losing money and making a 1 percent profit.

The Pennsylvania Fresh Food Financing Initiative benefitted from its vision and its good fortune—an enthusiastic and powerful political backer in Evans; a ready-made private partner in the Philadelphia-based Reinvestment Fund, a community development financial institution; the on-the-ground experience of The Food Trust; and some socially conscious grocers like Brown.

Since its creation nearly a decade ago, the Pennsylvania Fresh Food Financing Initiative has funded eighty-eight projects across the state, ranging from small greengrocers to farmers' markets and from natural-food cooperatives to large, full-service supermarkets. Typical of the way that the program has expanded to include all kinds of healthy food options is a $25,000 grant for refrigeration so that a small Korean grocer in Philadelphia's Logan section can now sell fresh foods. Officials claim that the funding helped to create or retain more than five thousand jobs while creating 1.67 million square feet of retail space.[3]

Equally important, the Pennsylvania experience provided The Food Trust with a template that it would seek to apply to other states, as publicity and concern over food deserts grew. The process involves two phases. In the first, The Food Trust uses grant money to create task forces, or food marketing groups, in targeted states. These task forces bring together stakeholders including public health officials and experts, grassroots activists, grocery executives, and political leaders—usually for the first time. The groups meet four or five times over the course of about a year, identify the areas most in need, and develop a plan of action. In most cases, the goal is a second phase similar to the Pennsylvania Fresh Food Financing Initiative—a public-private funding mechanism. The entire process takes several years before markets can be built or renovated.

—⌁— Expanding the Model

In the early 2000s, at the same time as The Food Trust's Supermarket Campaign was getting started, health policy experts were becoming increasingly alarmed by what Philadelphia activists had long been seeing in their neighborhoods: America was facing

a growing crisis of obesity and obesity-related illnesses, most
alarmingly among children. The greatest increases in obesity were
found in the same communities that had been largely abandoned
by the supermarket industry—those housing the urban and rural
poor, especially African Americans.

The Robert Wood Johnson Foundation's Support of The Food Trust

In 2003, shortly after Risa Lavizzo-Mourey became its president
and CEO, the Robert Wood Johnson Foundation made reversing
childhood obesity, especially among the poor, one of its strategic
priorities. In April 2007, it raised the ante by announcing a
commitment of $500 million to reverse the upward trend in
childhood obesity by 2015. The program staff at the Foundation
developed a wide-ranging strategy to address the environmental
factors leading to childhood obesity; increasing access to healthy,
affordable food through supermarkets and other outlets was a
component of this strategy.

The staff identified The Food Trust as an organization that
was ahead of the curve when it came to increasing access to healthy
food. Officials at the Foundation were impressed with both the
vision of The Food Trust and its methodical approach of bringing
together stakeholders. Judith Stavisky, a Foundation program
officer at the time, lived and frequently shopped in Philadelphia,
including at the Reading Terminal Market; she knew all about
The Food Trust's supermarket efforts and immediately saw the
potential for a partnership. "There was a sense of urgency but also
a sense that we had to do things thoughtfully," Stavisky recalls.

In 2004, the Foundation awarded a small grant to The Food
Trust to promote healthier food choices in corner stores. Two
years later, it made a grant of approximately $400,000 to replicate
the Pennsylvania model of supermarket development in Louisiana
and Illinois. In 2008, it awarded $475,000 to develop supermar-
kets in the Foundation's home state of New Jersey. Even as these
efforts were gaining steam, the Foundation increased it support,

awarding The Food Trust an additional $1.7 million in 2009 to develop supermarkets in low-income areas of eight states: Arizona, Georgia, Maryland, Massachusetts, Minnesota, Mississippi, Tennessee, and Texas. Then in 2012, the Foundation awarded $12 million to The Reinvestment Fund to administer funds for the New Jersey Food Access Initiative. The initiative, initially seeded by the New Jersey Economic Development Authority, is supporting the development of supermarkets and other sources of healthy food throughout the Foundation's home state, with The Food Trust playing a key role.

New York State's Healthy Food & Healthy Communities Fund

In New York State, The Food Trust partnered with the Low Income Investment Fund, Goldman Sachs, and others in establishing a $30 million fund for supermarket development. The Healthy Food & Healthy Communities Fund made it possible to develop supermarkets in communities with little access to healthy food, be they in the inner city or in the countryside. Just fifty miles north of New York City, for example, the small, leafy village of Highland Falls—wedged between steep mountains and a majestic bend in the Hudson River and abutting the historic gates of the United States Military Academy at West Point—is not a place that you would think of as a desert in any traditional use of the word. But when a moderately sized, rundown Key Food supermarket finally closed in 2009, Highland Falls joined the growing list of American food deserts.

For more than two years, residents with cars planned out the trek "over the mountain"—up steep winding roads to a large Walmart some eleven miles away, while village officials scrambled to offer van services to a large community of senior citizens. The only local food options were a small deli or the McDonald's and pizza joint near the entrance to the military academy. It is no wonder, then, that the October 2011 grand opening of the MyTown Marketplace was welcomed in Highland Falls not so much as just another store but as an oasis.

Albert Rodriguez, a veteran of the large food markets in the Bronx who had moved to the Hudson Valley with his wife, Lisa Berrios, a decade earlier, saw an opportunity at the sixteen-thousand-square-foot market that the larger chains had missed. They decided to buy it. Now the couple practically lives inside the brightly lit, completely overhauled store—there's a big couch in the office. Its large wooden bins, hand-built by Rodriguez and a friend, now teem with produce including apples from nearby farms. But the energetic couple never could have pulled off the expensive overhaul of the store without the start-up financing from the New York Healthy Food & Healthy Communities Fund.

Their vision for Highland Falls had encountered deep skepticism from banks, food wholesalers, and others. "When you're out of the business, nobody wants to do anything with you," Rodriguez says. After the couple learned of New York's new financing fund, they quickly applied and theirs was the first project approved. It was the public-private partnership that "made it happen," Rodriguez says. Besides giving Rodriguez and Berrios access to low-interest loan financing, the grant money allowed them to refurbish the store, which now glistens with bright lighting, sleek shelves, and even a freshly paved parking lot.

Berrios is practically giddy as she shows off an entire aisle devoted to gluten-free foods or the shiny walls that her husband put up, but nothing gives her more pride than the large produce corner near the front of the store. "The old store didn't have any of these things ... ginger, shallots, dried red chili peppers, tarragon," she says. "Everything just moves," her husband adds, holding up variety packages of vegetables sliced for grilling. "We don't have much waste at all. Packages like these, I can't keep them on the shelf."

The U.S. Government's Healthy Food Financing Initiative

Childhood obesity has become a front-burner national issue, boosted by the decision of First Lady Michelle Obama to make it her signature issue. Mrs. Obama invited ShopRite's Jeff Brown as one of her guests at the 2010 State of the Union address. In July 2011, the White House announced that leading retailers such as Walgreens, Walmart, and SuperValu had agreed to open at least 1,500 new stores in food deserts, home to as many as 9.5 million Americans.

In 2011, the federal government set out to implement a nationwide program patterned closely after The Food Trust's program in Pennsylvania. The White House's goal, which has been proposed in the last three budget cycles and is backed by proposed legislation in Congress, would create a Healthy Food Financing Initiative with roughly $285 million (in the latest version) to be administered by the Treasury Department, the Health and Human Services Department, and the Agriculture Department. That more ambitious plan has faltered on Capitol Hill, particularly after fiscal conservatism took root in the 2010 elections.

But the administration has been able to carve out smaller amounts to launch the Healthy Food Financing Initiative. In the fall of 2011, twenty-eight community-development programs received $35 million in grants from federal agencies for supermarkets and other healthy food projects. The administration's most recent plan takes a different approach, with $250 million in healthy food financing through the already existing New Markets Tax Credit Program. The various proposals in Washington offer the possibility of a major expansion in the type of program pioneered by The Food Trust.

—ᴍ— Implementing the Robert Wood Johnson Foundation-Funded Supermarket Campaign

The Food Trust's campaign to develop supermarkets in eight states, which is funded by the Robert Wood Johnson Foundation, began operating in 2010. Brian Lang, who directs the Supermarket Campaign, says that in trying to develop supermarkets in these states through the task force process, the campaign has run into a variety of hurdles. "For every state, there are a few issues," he notes. In a progressive, activist state such as Minnesota, for example, supermarket development must compete with a slew of other legislative priorities. In conservative states, the backlash that played out in the 2010 midterm elections makes any role for government-involved, taxpayer-funded solutions politically problematic. Here is how the project is playing out in a sampling of states.

Maryland

From the rough-hewn streets of Baltimore to the rural rolling hills on the state's western edge, officials have mapped a number of areas where statistics show a high rate of obesity and a paucity of supermarkets. One is a desolate neighborhood of Baltimore called Cherry Hill, where residents have little reason to hope that a modern supermarket like the Hudson Valley's MyTown will locate there any time in the near future.

Perched on a hilltop that overlooks Baltimore's skyscrapers but is geographically cut off by the Inner Harbor and an elevated stretch of I-95, Cherry Hill has not had a grocery store in years. As a result, the Baltimore City Health Department chose it as one of six locations for its online virtual supermarket, or Baltimarket. Here, two young staffers show up with a laptop once a week for three hours, taking grocery orders that will be forwarded to Santoni's, a popular supermarket several miles away; the orders will be delivered to Cherry Hill's public library the following day.

On this particular afternoon, Laura Fox, Baltimarket's coordinator, arrives at the library at 12:30. Spreading a bright red-and-white plastic cloth over a front table, she sets out today's sample—a cabbage salad spiked with raisins and pineapple—in small plastic cups. Soon Fox is joined by one of the regulars, Betty Bailey—"Miss Betty," as Fox calls her. Now sixty-five, Bailey lives around the corner, alone and unemployed since she lost a job as a cashier three years ago. Before she found out about the Baltimarket program, Bailey had to call her daughter in suburban

Glen Burnie for a ride to a supermarket. Now she comes in every two weeks and orders roughly $40 worth of groceries each time, roughly equal to how much she receives in food stamps. Spurred on by a $10 discount for healthy items on the initial order, Bailey says she finds herself more likely to order fruits than before, especially blueberries. "My great-grandson likes to reach over and pick them up while I'm eating them," she says, laughing. "He's eating them faster than I am and he's not even two, so he's learning how to eat healthy."

Elsewhere in Maryland, Larry Hentz, a business development specialist in the Prince George's County Economic Development Corporation and a key member of the Maryland supermarket task force, admits he stumbled onto the issue when a Safeway store serving Hillcrest Heights, a middle-class, predominantly black Maryland suburb of Washington, D.C., abruptly announced it was shutting down in thirty days. Safeway officials told Hentz the store had been losing money for a decade and that the chain had found it impossible to make a profit on the East Coast unless a store is at least forty-five thousand square feet, or nearly double the footprint in Hillcrest Heights. Hentz called a meeting of community residents. "There was a lot of anger," he says. "People said, 'Where am I going to get my essentials?'" That's when Hentz realized that a supermarket was more vital to the everyday life of a neighborhood than any other development project he'd worked on before.

After that, he worked with local churches to launch a van service to the nearest open supermarket several miles away while he scoured the eastern seaboard for a successful urban supermarket company looking to expand. Hentz learned that the owner of Evergreen Supermarket had been eyeing the D.C. region, hoping to develop a new chain of small grocery stores that would complement the county's larger supermarkets. Hentz promised the owner that he could streamline the elaborate approval process to allow for an opening at Thanksgiving and the more profitable holiday season, and he devoted much of his workday toward achieving that target. The Evergreen Supermarket in Hillcrest Heights opened on November 23, 2011—the day before Thanksgiving.

Arizona

In Arizona, The Food Trust and its allies decided the political situation was too toxic to move forward with the task force process. "Folks whom we could usually count on to be with us in an advocacy campaign are busy trying to put out other fires," says The Food Trust's Lang. "Like trying to get funding restored for children's health insurance." So The Food Trust elected to work with a supermarket company called Bashas', which operates grocery stores on Indian reservations in Arizona. Officials agreed that the fastest and simplest way to increase healthy eating among rural Native Americans is to increase offerings of fresh fruits and vegetables and lower-calorie products in Bashas' stores. The healthier product lines will be aggressively marketed through in-store marketing such as colorful displays, and the impact on diet and health will be compared to outcomes at five control stores.

Mississippi

Mississippi poses unusual challenges. For one thing, the state lacks a grocer's trade association, which in most other states has been a key player in The Food Trust's efforts. Perhaps even more important, the very character of the food-access problem is different in Mississippi—one of America's poorest states, where poverty in rural communities is widespread. According to Sandra Shelson of The Partnership for a Healthy Mississippi and one of the leaders of the state's task force effort, while their urban counterparts often buy food in corner stores or *bodegas*, Mississippi's rural poor typically shop instead in convenience stores. "They are these little hole-in-the-wall places where a lot of people go to get their food, but the prices are higher," says Shelson, lamenting that the aisles of these small stores are typically lined with every manner of sugary drinks and fatty foods. Meanwhile, there is usually a counter where such high-fat staples as fried chicken and potato logs are served to customers with limited public-assistance budgets.

The Mississippi task force also faces a problem with density, Shelson says. "Many of these isolated communities are impractical sites for a large well-stocked supermarket." Much of the group's discussion, therefore, has focused on how farmers' markets could augment the convenience-store diet while tapping into the agricultural bounty of a crop-producing state.

Shelson also notes—as have Supermarket Campaign task force members in other states—that the experience of bringing together public health officials with grocers and food wholesalers has been a valuable learning experience for everyone involved. Shelson is optimistic that the task force's recommendations and its subsequent promotion of them will result in public backing for new markets, even in an era of Tea Party–inspired fiscal conservatism. The idea would be to play up job creation, since economic development is one role for government that Mississippians have continued to support. "We have to be very strategic. The public health perspective is not where a lot of people are coming from," Shelson says.

Tennessee

"It's not in the portfolio of the health department to be speaking about small business development," says Tennessee task force member Kenneth Robinson, a physician and public health policy adviser to the mayor of Shelby County, which includes Memphis. Speaking as the Tennessee Grocery Access Task Force was nearing completion of its work, Robinson says it was a new experience bridging public health worries with the issues and concerns of a for-profit industry.

He believes that the discussions between the competing stakeholders may lead to some innovative solutions. For example, grocery representatives told the task force that it is difficult to stock fresh produce because of the uneven demand created when so much benefit money is distributed around the first of the month. The group may recommend that Tennessee stagger payments so that supermarkets can expect a more dependable stream of customers. Robinson says that the task force is also looking at how to encourage food stamp (now known as SNAP) clients to use their benefits to purchase fruits and vegetables.

Boston, Massachusetts

Ronn Garry, one of the third-generation owners of Tropical Foods in Boston's impoverished Roxbury section, has an ambitious plan to expand the bustling market that his grandfather, a political refugee who fled Fidel Castro's Cuba, started in 1974 as a small corner shop called "El Platanero," or "The Banana Man." But Garry's proposal to build a modern twenty-thousand-square-foot market on two acres in what is now the dusty parking lot of his current property has been held up by bureaucratic red tape for close to six years. "Unless you're one of the big guys, the city doesn't really help you out," he says. Because of his concerns, Garry was an enthusiastic participant in the Massachusetts task force that was established through the Supermarket Campaign.

Indeed, Tropical Foods seems to be bursting at the seams on a spring morning early in the month when many in Roxbury have received their benefit payments. Lines at the cashiers run to ten-deep. Other customers circle past bright Caribbean-themed murals on their way to the store's fresh produce department, which is not large but is well stocked with vegetables that are popular with shoppers from the islands or Latin America—a rarity at chain supermarkets. "*Malanga, malanga, malanga,*" one Spanish-speaking customer mutters with delight as she passes a bin overflowing with the brown shaggy root that is a staple in places like Cuba and Puerto Rico. "We reflect the community that we serve," Garry says proudly.

Despite Tropical Foods' expansion woes, the store still offers Roxbury residents substantially more square feet of supermarket than exists in the urban core of Springfield, western Massachusetts' largest city. That's why activist Frank Robinson, from Partners for a Healthier Community, raced to Boston on a recent afternoon to attend the final meeting of the state task force. Hoping that the momentum from the Supermarket Campaign and more governmental support would lead to the supermarket he's been promoting for over five years, "I think the task force has raised awareness around the issue. Robinson says, It's created the beginning of mobilization."

For roughly two hours, Robinson, Garry, and about thirty others from an array of community and food-industry groups, plus state government aides—most of them strangers to one another little more than a year earlier—sat in a plush wood-paneled conference room at the Federal Reserve Bank of Boston and spoke of a shared vision for more supermarkets and healthier residents. The draft of the task force's final report contained a number of recommendations, including a commitment to partnerships for workforce training, affordable transit options, and giving priority to supermarkets and other healthy food stores in the urban planning process. But the most important goal is also the one that will be the hardest to attain: creating a Fresh Food Financing Fund modeled after the public-private partnerships in Pennsylvania and New York. As the Robert Wood Johnson Foundation's grant money wound down in 2012, most of the other task forces created through The Food Trust were expected to call for similar funding mechanisms.

—⌇— Encountering—and Countering—Skepticism

In recent years, with the high-profile push from the federal government embracing the supermarket-development cause pioneered by The Food Trust, skeptics have emerged in the scientific and public health communities. They note that although many of the urban neighborhoods targeted by programs like the Supermarket Campaign may be "deserts" when it comes to affordable fruits and vegetables, they are also "food swamps" for "takeouts"—heavy on fast-food outlets, snack-laden corner stores, and takeout foods like fried chicken and burgers. These critics cite evidence that low-income Americans will continue to seek out foods that are high in fat and sugar—because less healthy, processed foods cost less and are heavily marketed by the food industry, and also because our bodies are genetically programmed to crave foods that are no longer good for us.

Advocacy groups like The Food Trust counter that an overwhelming preponderance of the research that has been done over two decades does suggest a strong link between access to a supermarket and better health outcomes. "We've collected one hundred thirty-two studies from the last twenty years," says the Food Trust's Yael Lehmann, "and every one shows a positive impact." She cites the studies of Akihiko Michimi as examples.

Michimi, an assistant professor at Western Kentucky University, studies relationships between geography and public health. Using extensive data on obesity and eating habits compiled from telephone surveys of U.S. citizens conducted by the Center for Disease Control and Prevention (CDC), Michimi and coresearcher Michael Wimberly initially noted a significant correlation between where people lived and their risk for obesity. They found a generally higher risk for obesity in rural areas, especially in the Midwest and South. Michimi and Wimberly decided to delve into the data to factor in the proximity to a large supermarket. What the researchers found, according to a 2010 report, was somewhat surprising: distance to a supermarket did not affect rural obesity rates, but made a difference in urban areas.[4]

"Distance to a supermarket really matters in the urban areas," Michimi says. He notes that transportation could be a factor, as residents of an urban food desert are less likely to own a car than their rural counterparts. "If you have enough income, you could still drive a couple of miles to the supermarket, but poor people in urban areas don't have this option." Still, Michimi admits there's a need for much more research into the complicated relationship between diet, supermarket access, and socioeconomic factors.

That is the chicken-or-egg conundrum. Do people fail to eat fruits and vegetables because there are no supermarkets nearby? Or are there no supermarkets nearby because people who live in urban food deserts prefer to eat processed food and fast food because it is cheaper, tastes better, or is more appealing? The latter alternative offers profit-driven grocery stores little incentive to set up shop.

In the spring of 2012, with the national obesity crisis in the news and with Food Trust-led task forces working to create funding mechanisms and governmental support for new supermarkets, two academic studies made news by suggesting that the link between grocery access and a healthy diet was at best overstated and possibly nonexistent. Because the concept of "food deserts" had become so entrenched in the public health conversation, these contrarian reports hit the front page of *The New York Times*, ensuring national controversy.[5]

One paper, based on research from the RAND Corporation and published in the *American Journal of Preventive Medicine* in February 2012, analyzed self-reported data on weight, height, and diet from roughly thirteen thousand California schoolchildren, and correlated the children's addresses with nearby supermarkets and other food outlets.[6] One of the researchers, Roland Sturm, reported he could find no connection between childhood obesity and proximity to a market.

Meanwhile, Helen Lee, a researcher at the Public Policy Institute of California, also used a large pool of data—from a national survey of nearly eight thousand children—along with mapping information about the location and size of food outlets. Lee reported that while lower-income neighborhoods had more fast-food restaurants and convenience stores, as expected, they also had a higher density of supermarkets and other large food outlets than more affluent zip codes did.

Both researchers told the *Times* that the evidence suggests that lack of access to healthy food is not a primary cause of obesity. Sturm told the newspaper that poor urban neighborhoods often have an array of food outlets including fast-food restaurants and takeouts, and should be called food swamps—not food deserts. He said that his study did not find a correlation between where children lived, nearby food outlets, and obesity.

Barry Popkin, a professor of nutrition at the University of North Carolina, is a leading skeptic when it comes to blaming obesity on lack of access to fruits and vegetables. He chaired an Institute of Medicine and National Research Council committee that reviewed the available research on food access and community health, including several studies from the United Kingdom. The National Academy of Sciences panel concluded that "food retail is only one component of the total food environment that affects how people eat" and that evidence that a supermarket in the neighborhood leads to healthier eating is lacking.[7] Popkin says that poor urban residents typically find that the best produce is out of their price range. Furthermore, they have a fundamental lack of knowledge about how to prepare healthy meals or even what comprises a beneficial diet. He also believes the current obesity crisis is largely a creation of human beings' calorie-craving biology and rapid advances in food-industry technology. "It takes a lot to change a diet," Popkin says. "It isn't just having carrots in the front of a store."

The backlash led, not surprisingly, to a strong response from advocates for supermarket access. For one thing, experts noted that in attempting to develop large data pools, the contrarian researchers had used questionable methodology. Allison Karpyn, director of research and evaluation for The Food Trust, questions the reliability of self-reporting by teenagers about their diet, which was at the core of the RAND study. She also notes that the Public Policy Institute of California study had started out with a much larger group of kids—roughly twenty thousand (before whittling the sample down to eight thousand kids)—and that children who stayed in one location and were included in the final study tended to come from higher socioeconomic households. That could skew the findings.

But the most significant criticism of the research of the super-market skeptics is that they are attacking a "straw man," because groups such as The Food Trust have never stated that access to healthy food alone was enough to change health outcomes in poor or isolated communities. "Supermarkets are part—and only part—of the solution to a deeply rooted and complex prob-lem," says Jamie Bussel, the program officer at the Robert Wood Johnson Foundation who oversees the Foundation's grants to The Food Trust. "That's why the Foundation has taken a broad approach to reducing childhood obesity and why The Food Trust supports bodegas and small grocery stores as well as supermar-kets and works in rural as well as urban areas." Chicago-based researcher Mari Gallagher, whose work helped popularize the term "food desert," wrote, "To my knowledge, no one of any credibility has ever suggested that access was the entire solution or that anything involving the complicated relationship between diet and health is simple."[8]

Experts like The Food Trust's Karpyn say another problem is that most skeptics' research takes a secondhand approach of mapping public health and store locations and inferring linkages from large samples of data. "I'm as frustrated as anyone that we don't have better studies," says Karpyn.

The Food Trust and its supporters are awaiting the results of firsthand studies directly addressing the question of whether and how the arrival of a well-stocked supermarket affects eating habits and health. The researchers hope to gain significantly more knowledge when two studies in particular, both taking place in The Food Trust's home state of Pennsylvania, are completed.

The first is a RAND study that involves surveys conducted before and after a supermarket opens in an urban, low-income neighborhood of Pittsburgh. The opening is currently scheduled for spring 2013. An almost identical study is partially completed in Philadelphia, where a Penn State researcher designed a project around the reopening of a supermarket in North Philadelphia's Progress Plaza, an iconic development with roots in the civil rights movement of the 1960s. Both studies involve extensive research on neighborhood residents, their eating habits, and their health about six to nine months before and after the opening of the store.

—⚉— Waging Battle One Kale Salad at a Time

When policy experts look at the frontlines of the urban obesity war, they see well-stocked supermarkets as one of many battles. They look at activists like Joyce Smith, the executive director of Operation ReachOut Southwest in Baltimore. When Smith moved back into Southwest Baltimore about two decades ago, her native neighborhood was so overtaken by abandoned factories, boarded-up homes, drug-dealing, and gun violence that it would become the setting for David Simon's 1997 book *The Corner*, which in turn would inspire an HBO mini-series. In real life, The Corner at Fayette and Monroe is now largely cleaned up, and Smith realizes that more of her neighbors are dying from burgers than from bullets. Her current crusade for healthy eating was inspired by 2008 data from the Baltimore City Health Department, which revealed that the life expectancy of residents of Smith's corner of the city is twenty years shorter than that of residents of an upscale neighborhood called Roland Park.

"I noticed that people were eating to address hunger," says Smith, speaking at her office inside a Southwest Baltimore community center. "They weren't eating to address health." So when a new Food Depot, one of just two supermarkets owned and operated by a longtime Baltimore food wholesaler, opened two years ago in an abandoned location in the nearby Westside Shopping Center, Smith worked with local groups like the Center for a Livable Future at Johns Hopkins University to make the retailer responsive to the community. The store's owner has launched a shuttle bus service and led "Shopping Matters" tours to teach residents skills like finding the best price for produce or identifying whole-grain breads. Smith also continues to operate a small farmers' market at the MARC rail station in West Baltimore on Saturday afternoons. That gives Southwest Baltimore residents another healthy food option.

It also gives the talkative grandmother a chance to do what she does best: evangelize for a healthier lifestyle. Smith says that access to fruits and vegetables means more when urban residents understand the consequences of their food choices. She asks her neighbors if they have a relative with diabetes or who died young of a heart attack, and she tries to explain it was probably a consequence of what they ate. In a world where celebrations are often equated with a bucket of fried chicken, Smith raises eyebrows by bringing fresh greens, or water instead of soda. "I remember I made a kale salad at one of our celebrations and this lady came up and said, 'Miss Smith, the kale is cold!' I said, 'It's a kale salad; it's supposed to be cold.' She'd never seen a kale salad."

Smith knows instinctively what many public health experts have come to realize over the years: U.S. communities need markets with fresh produce and whole-wheat bread, but that is just one piece of the puzzle, along with education, more effective anti-poverty programs, and other solutions. "It has to be multiple pronged," Smith says. "Having access is part of it, but it's also changing habits." It's a battle she wages one kale salad at a time.

Notes

1. Ferguson, B. and Abell, B. "The Urban Grocery Store Gap." *Economic Development Commentary*, Winter 1998, 6–14.
2. U.S. Department of Agriculture, Economic Research Service. *Access to Affordable and Nutritious Food: Understanding Food Deserts and Their Consequences*, June 2009.
3. The Reinvestment Fund, The Pennsylvania Fresh Food Financing Initiative. *Providing Healthy Food Choices to Pennsylvania Communities*, 2007, p. 4.

4. Michimi, A. and Wimberly, C. "Associations of Supermarket Accessibility with Obesity and Fruit and Vegetable Consumption in the Conterminous United States." *International Journal of Health Geographics*, 2010, 9, 49.

5. Kolata, G. "Studies Question the Pairing of Food Deserts and Obesity." *New York Times*, April 18, 2012, p. A1.

6. An, R. and Sturm, R. "School and Residential Neighborhood Food Environment and Diet among California Youth." *American Journal of Preventive Medicine*, February 2012, 129–135.

7. National Academy of Sciences. *The Public Health Effects of Food Deserts: Workshop Summary*, www.nap.edu/catalog/12623.html, 2009.

8. Gallagher, M. "Response to 'Studies Question Pairing of Food Deserts and Obesity,'" http://marigallagher.com/site_media/dynamic/project_files /RESPONSE_NYT_FOODDESERTS-OBESITY.pdf.

CHAPTER 11

Populating Population Health

The Health & Society Scholars and the Young Epidemiology Scholars Programs

Tony Proscio

Editors' Introduction

The very first grants made by the newly minted Robert Wood Johnson Foundation were for scholarships to enable needy students—minorities, women, and people from rural areas—to attend medical school. These marked the first in a long line of scholarship and fellowship programs to improve the qualifications, credibility, and diversity of those working in the health and health care fields.[1] In fact, although the Foundation takes pride in its strategic planning, clearly stated tactical goals, and quantitatively measurable outcomes, a substantial percentage of its expenditures—some $765 million, or approximately 9 percent, over the past forty years—has gone to fellowships and scholarships whose value, though not so easily measurable in the short run, is indisputable.

   The Foundation has used its fellowship and scholarship programs to strengthen fields to which it has given priority. A list of the fields and programs is provided in the appendix to this introduction.

   In the late 1990s, in conjunction with dividing its programming into health and health care, the Foundation began focusing attention on the emerging field of population health (that is, the health of large numbers of people, as contrasted with individuals). Following its practice of seeding academic research in areas that it deems important, the Foundation launched two new fellowship programs to strengthen population health research: the Robert Wood Johnson Foundation Health & Society Scholars and the Young Epidemiology Scholars. In this chapter, Tony Proscio, a journalist and consultant to foundations and nonprofit organizations, examines these programs—their derivation, their activities, their recipients, and their significance.

Appendix: The Robert Wood Johnson Foundation's Fellowship and Scholarship Programs

Government, Academic, and Nonprofit Health Policy Leadership

- Robert Wood Johnson Foundation Clinical Scholars Program (1972–present)[2]

- Robert Wood Johnson Foundation Health Policy Fellows (1973–present)[3]

Health Services and Policy Research[4]

- Faculty Fellowships in Health Care Finance (1984–1994)

- Scholars in Health Policy Research Program (1991–present)

- Investigator Awards in Health Policy Research (1991–present)

- Robert Wood Johnson Foundation Center for Health Policy at the University of New Mexico (2007–present)

- Robert Wood Johnson Foundation Center for Health Policy at Meharry Medical College (2009–present)

Nursing[5]

- Nurse Faculty Fellowship Program (1975–1982)

- Clinical Nurse Scholars (1982–1991)

- Robert Wood Johnson Foundation Executive Nurse Fellows (1997–present)

- Robert Wood Johnson Foundation Nursing and Health Policy Collaborative at the University of New Mexico (2007–present)

- Robert Wood Johnson Foundation Nurse Faculty Scholars (2012–present)

Diversity

- Preprofessional Minority Programs (1974–1992)

- Harold Amos Medical Faculty Development Program (1983–present)[6]

- Summer Medical and Dental Education Program (1987–present)[7]

- Health Professions Partnership Initiative (1994–2006)[8]

- New Connections: Increasing Diversity of the Robert Wood Johnson Foundation Programming (2005–present)

Primary Care Physicians

- Primary Care Residency Program (1973–1981)
- Family Practice Faculty Fellowships Program (1976–1988)
- General Pediatric Academic Development Program (1976–1988)
- Generalist Physician Faculty Scholars (1992–1999)
- Generalist Provider Research Initiative (1993–1999)
- Robert Wood Johnson Foundation Physician Faculty Scholars (2006–2012)

Dental Research

- Dental Services Research Scholars Program (1982–1990)[9]

Public Health

- Public Health Pipeline Program (1997–2006)
- Public Health Informatics Fellows Training Program (2004–2011)
- Public Health Workforce: Public Health Nursing (2011–present)

Community Health Leadership

- Ladder to Leadership: Developing the Next Generation of Community Health Leaders (2007–2013)

Notes

1. See Isaacs, S. L., Sandy, L. G., and Schroeder, S. A. "Improving the Health Care Workforce: Perspectives from Twenty-Four Years' Experience." *To Improve Health and Health Care 1997: The Robert Wood Johnson Foundation Anthology*. San Francisco: Jossey-Bass, 1997.
2. See Showstack, J., Anderson Rothman, A., Leviton, L. C., and Sandy, L. G. "The Robert Wood Johnson Clinical Scholars Program." *To Improve Health and Health Care: The Robert Wood Johnson Foundation Anthology*, Vol. VII. San Francisco: Jossey-Bass, 2004.
3. See Frank, R. S. "The Health Policy Fellowships Program." *To Improve Health and Health Care: The Robert Wood Johnson Foundation Anthology*, Vol. V. San Francisco: Jossey-Bass, 2002.

4. See Colby, D. C. "Building Health Policy Research in the Social Sciences." *To Improve Health and Health Care: The Robert Wood Johnson Foundation Anthology*, Vol. VI. San Francisco: Jossey-Bass, 2003.

5. See Newbergh, C. "The Robert Wood Johnson Foundation's Commitment to Nursing." *To Improve Health and Health Care: The Robert Wood Johnson Foundation Anthology*, Vol. VIII. San Francisco: Jossey-Bass, 2005.

6. This was originally the Minority Medical Faculty Program. See Lowe, J. and Pechura, C. "The Robert Wood Johnson Foundation's Commitment to Increasing Minorities in the Health Professions." *To Improve Health and Health Care: The Robert Wood Johnson Foundation Anthology*, Vol. VII. San Francisco: Jossey-Bass, 2004.

7. This was originally the Minority Medical Education Program. See Bergeisen, L. and Cantor, J. "The Minority Medical Education Program." *To Improve Health and Health Care 2000: The Robert Wood Johnson Foundation Anthology*. San Francisco: Jossey-Bass, 2000.

8. Note 6, op. cit.

9. See Brodeur, P. "Improving Dental Care." *To Improve Health and Health Care 2001: The Robert Wood Johnson Foundation Anthology*. San Francisco: Jossey-Bass, 2001.

—⁓— **B**y the end of the current decade, public health systems in the United States will face a shortage of more than a quarter-million skilled employees, according to a 2008 study by the Association of Schools of Public Health.[1] Yet even this estimate, focusing mainly on professionals with health care or public health credentials, probably understates the real talent gap. Promoting and protecting the health of large populations—reducing injury and preventable illness, instilling healthy behavior, identifying and eliminating hazards, and sharpening public policy that affects people's health and well-being—is too broad a mission to be limited solely to graduates of medical, nursing, and public health schools.

Increasingly, the challenges of public health—more broadly understood in recent years as *population* health—call for an interdisciplinary network of natural and social scientists, humanities scholars, health professionals, specialists in management and finance, and policy experts, as well as people from the fields more traditionally found in a typical government public health agency. But not only are there too few representatives from most of these fields currently working on health-related issues, the goal of forming a true network among them is still largely a dream. A genuinely interdisciplinary *field* of population health[2] would encompass multiple centers of cross-disciplinary research and innovation, along with a frontline workforce that routinely combines people of widely differing skills and backgrounds; and it would feature a web of steady, open channels of communication among the many areas of expertise. Some outstanding public health organizations, working groups, and projects have been known to exhibit some of these qualities, but those remain relatively small and noteworthy exceptions in a world still dominated by firmly bounded scholarly disciplines and hermetically separate professions.

One critical part of the problem is that many people with relevant interests and talent—budding sociologists, economists, anthropologists, public policy experts, business managers and financiers, urban planners, and an array of natural scientists, among others—do not think of themselves as candidates for a career in population health. Many may not even know such a field exists, and others may simply be unable to imagine how their skills would fit into the mosaic of different disciplines and backgrounds that such a field would need. And in truth, there are plenty of influences to discourage them.

Especially en route to an academic career, degree candidates and postdoctoral scholars are often actively dissuaded from pursuing research outside the confines of their own disciplines. It is within those disciplines, after all, that the rules of entry and promotion tend to be written—rules that govern advanced degree programs, fellowships and residencies, scholarly publications, and ultimately the competition for tenure. Gatekeepers of established disciplines may look askance on work that ventures into what, by orthodox standards, amounts to alien territory. "Particularly in more prestigious universities, with more of a research agenda," says David Kindig, professor emeritus at the University of Wisconsin School of Medicine and Public Health, "departments tend to see the world through their own lens, and it tends to be within their traditional disciplinary boundaries."

—⌇— Investing in a Diversity of Talent

Drawing more disciplines and a greater variety of expertise into health scholarship has been an interest of the Robert Wood Johnson Foundation for most of its history. The earliest and best known of the Foundation's efforts to develop the "human capital" of individual talent and leadership has been its flagship Robert Wood Johnson Foundation Clinical Scholars program, which annually provides two years of study for roughly two dozen young clinicians to broaden their knowledge of such fields as health services, epidemiology, economics, law, biostatistics, management, and ethics to enable them to become leaders in the field. Incubated at the Carnegie Corporation of New York and The Commonwealth Fund, the Clinical Scholars program moved to the Robert Wood Johnson Foundation shortly after its founding in 1972, and has flourished there for four decades.

In 1973, its second year of operation, the Foundation created the Health Policy Fellows program, which initially sent health professionals, and later behavioral and social scientists, to Washington every year to work on health policy issues in Congress or the Executive Branch. Then in 1991 the Scholars in Health Policy Research Program was launched, aiming more specifically at academic research on health policy by recent PhDs in economics, political science, and sociology. An even broader effort followed a year later, when the Investigator Awards in Health Policy Research began offering up to three years of support for young researchers or eminent scholars from virtually any discipline.[3]

These programs tended to focus more on health *care*, both practice and policy, than on the broader and more fundamental question of societal health. But the Foundation's mission called for efforts to improve both *health* and health care. Beginning in the late 1990s, the Foundation's president, Steven Schroeder, began taking steps within the organization to right the balance between the two halves of the mission. In 1999, with the Foundation reorganized into a Health Group and a Health Care Group, he hired J. Michael McGinnis, a physician and influential federal health official who had served under four presidents, as senior vice president and founding director of the newly formed Health Group. It was no coincidence that some of McGinnis's earlier research and writing had helped to demonstrate that medical care is only one, and perhaps the least powerful, of several types of determinants of health, among them genetic, behavioral, social, and environmental factors.

"We can even make a quantitative estimate of the relative importance of each of these," McGinnis said. "But what's important is not so much the individual factors as the *interaction among them*, the intersections of these various domains."

His work at the Foundation, therefore, focused on developing initiatives that drew on a variety of interlocking fields to promote population health—for example, a group of programs under the umbrella of Active Living, designed to integrate multiple lines of effort—research, community development, leadership training, and networking—to encourage physical activity and develop a field around it. And he sought ways of cultivating leaders from multiple disciplines and forming cross-pollinating relationships among them. Eventually these would form, in his words, "the infrastructure of a fully functioning field."

To help populate that field—not only to enrich it with outstanding individuals but also to galvanize institutions and networks—McGinnis proposed two new individual-awards programs, fundamentally different in scope and design from any the Foundation had attempted before.

The first of these new programs, known as Health & Society Scholars, had some strategic roots in the earlier Investigator Awards model: not limited to particular disciplines, it was intended to recruit rising stars from many fields. But this time, the purpose went beyond advancing individual careers or specific lines of inquiry; now the goal was also, and more particularly, to expand interdisciplinary research into ways of fostering a healthier society—to "increase the nation's effectiveness in addressing the multiple underlying determinants of health and disease," in the words of an early strategy memo. Success would therefore be measured not only by the amount of important work being done by outstanding people; it would also be measured by how much the principle of cross-disciplinary collaboration had penetrated the institutions where those people studied and worked, and ultimately how much it had penetrated American health scholarship as a whole.

The second new human capital effort bore virtually no resemblance to any previous Robert Wood Johnson initiative. The Young Epidemiology Scholars, or YES, program offered college scholarships of varying amounts to high school students who excelled in a national research competition. By investigating some issue in population health—the definition of eligible topics was intentionally broad—students could win anywhere from $1,000 to $50,000 toward their college tuition. Sixty regional finalists each year also got a trip to Washington, D.C., where they spent time with one another, met influential figures in epidemiology and public health, and presented their projects before elite panels of judges.

The two programs have contributed in different ways to what Pamela Russo, the senior program officer who oversees the programs at the Foundation, describes as "the Health Group's unifying theme: the social and environmental determinants of health, and the multiple sectors that have to be involved to formulate effective health policies." Both programs seek to inspire outstanding people, at different but relatively early points on the career ladder, to think broadly about health—and, armed with the tools of many different intellectual fields, to approach the health of whole populations from multiple points of view.

—∾— The Health & Society Scholars

The first of the two programs began with a planning phase in 2001 to select six participating universities and to settle on the basic structure, requirements, and curricula. In 2002, the first eighteen fellowships were awarded with $31 million from the Foundation for the first five years of operation (due to the drop in the Foundation's endowment in 2007–2008, the number of scholarships was reduced to twelve per year beginning in 2011). Between 2002 and 2013, the Foundation allotted more than $92 million. Most of that amount pays for stipends for participating scholars and support to the six universities, with the remainder paying for management by a national program office.

Each year, the Health & Society Scholars are selected to spend two years at one of the participating universities. Most of the scholars are postdoctoral students, though a few are in early stages of academic careers. During their scholarship years, they take courses, participate in interdisciplinary seminars, and pursue research with the guidance or collaboration of resident faculty. They also work closely with peers from other departments, either in self-organized collaborations or through formal interdisciplinary working groups. They benefit from mentoring by senior faculty members, not only on the substance of their scholarship, but on leadership, career development, competition for research grants, and ways of thriving when they return to regular academic life, which for most will be in traditional disciplines and departments.

"It's essentially a two-year immersion in interdisciplinary culture," says the program's national codirector, Christine Almy Bachrach. "Through much of that time, you're working alongside people who have been trained in a very different way from you. And that's a crucial part of the program, because a great deal of the challenge of interdisciplinary work involves human skills: How do you listen to and communicate with someone whose scientific frames of reference have been developed in ways that are foreign to you? How do you get on the same page with that person and speak the same language? How do you combine your methods and approach to research with theirs?"

The six participating institutions are Columbia University, Harvard University, the University of California at San Francisco and at Berkeley (a joint program links the two campuses), and the universities of Michigan, Pennsylvania, and Wisconsin-Madison. They were selected partly for their commitment to cultivating a fertile cross-disciplinary environment and partly for their ability to support that commitment with faculty and programs that can bridge the human, cultural, and intellectual divides among disciplines. Each of the six sites receives $1.1 million a year to administer the program, including the payment of an annual stipend of $80,000, plus some expenses and fringe benefits, to each scholar. The grant also includes $125,000 per site to help the universities strengthen their research in population health and to support the training of faculty and scholars.[4] Program faculty at the universities use this money to promote work on population health across their campuses and to award small competitive grants to Health & Society Scholars and other students or faculty. These grants help recipients develop promising population-health research that often leads to larger outside funding.

"These were universities that had identified themselves as wanting and needing to expand their interdisciplinary work on the determinants of health and health disparities, all critical to achieving population health," says the program's other codirector, Jo Ivey Boufford, president of The New York Academy of Medicine. "And at the same time, they also had some strengths to build on. Some had farther to go than others, but all of them had made this basic commitment and had ideas about how to achieve it." At each site, the program typically coalesced around what Boufford describes as "a core set of faculty, the mentors for the scholars, who were the nucleus, in a sense," of the interdisciplinary network interested in issues related to population health. "Then you'd have a next ring of faculty who agreed to be available, come to seminars, give talks—they were more loosely affiliated, but they were involved. And other relationships would begin to extend outward from those."

An essential hypothesis behind the program was that as the circle of affiliation widened, and as people closer to the nucleus became more deeply committed to it, the interdisciplinary climate would improve. The frequency of interaction would begin to create a cohesive enterprise, a hub of cross-disciplinary work that would have identity and purpose beyond the Robert Wood Johnson Foundation initiative. To test this hypothesis and track progress at each campus, the program conducted a social network analysis that mapped the networks of participating departments, centers, and programs at the start and then again eight years later. Connecting lines showed collaborations under way in 2002 and 2010, respectively. "The results," says Boufford, "were pretty spectacular." Sociograms showing one typical university's progress looked like this:

BEFORE

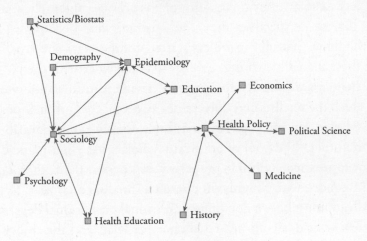

AFTER

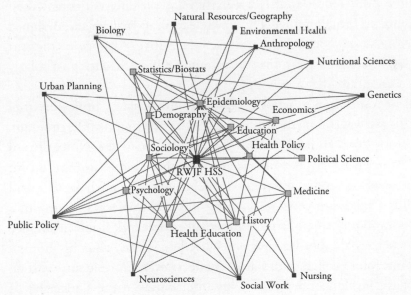

It seemed, according to Boufford, that the program's gravitational pull was working exactly as its designers had hoped—at least so far. Not only were more faculty members from more departments drawn to work with one another and with the Health & Society Scholars, but the quality of the scholars themselves, and the diverse perspectives they could bring, were becoming part of the draw. "Faculty members started competing," she says, "to get these incredible young scholars to come work with them."

Scholars are selected for each site based on advance interviews in which the finalists and universities assess the "fit" of their possible relationship and begin to envision how each would contribute to the other. The pool of applicant scholars has risen markedly, from approximately 150 in the early years to more than 300 for the 2011 cohort, with roughly 50 chosen as finalists each year. Every applicant must have a doctorate or terminal professional degree in a relevant field, significant research experience, and the ability to articulate a clear connection between their research interests and important issues in population health. Finalists interview at up to three different sites, after which they and the universities rank their interest in one another. The final selection and pairings are designed to ensure a good fit. By the time scholars arrive on campus at the start of the academic year, they are usually well matched to the scholarly community they are joining.

José Pagán, a labor economist and business professor from Texas, was among those selected for the first round of the program, from 2003 through 2005. He was drawn to the University of Pennsylvania, where some faculty members were examining health disparities among different ethnic groups. Pagán chose to spend his scholarship years researching the health effects of living in a community where large numbers of people lack health insurance (such as the border town of McAllen, Texas, near his home), and found evidence of harmful effects even on residents who do have insurance. Because of his interactions at the University of Pennsylvania, he says, "I'm a totally different person in the way I think about problems and the way I look at the world."

At Penn, all scholars participate in a general seminar in health and society and in a biweekly seminar on their work in progress, where they are exposed to one another's current research and the work of faculty members from several departments and disciplines. They also typically work in multidisciplinary teams on their own research projects, an experience that Pagán describes as "learning to think in a different language ... You're forced to think in the languages of many other fields, from biology to chemistry to urban planning to economics. That forces you to examine your research questions much more carefully and from more angles, knowing you have to communicate your ideas with people in other disciplines. You spend a lot of time in those two years distilling your ideas for that purpose."

But the program's influence on Pagán's later career extended beyond his intellectual interests and research. Individual mentoring and exposure to the work of university schools and departments also opened a critical window onto how multidisciplinary projects work—how they can be funded, how successful centers of interdisciplinary research are organized and managed, and how to retain credibility in one's own discipline while working across intellectual boundaries. After his time at the University of Pennsylvania, he returned to The University of Texas–Pan American and organized a new Institute for Population Health Policy, drawing on the insights and knowledge he had gained at the University of Pennsylvania.

"I wouldn't have been able to do that," he says, "without the networking and mentoring and learning in my two years at Penn—plus all the contacts with people at other sites. I spent a lot of time looking around and seeing how people did what they did. Why were the Penn people so successful getting interdisciplinary grants? How did they put together large projects? How do they structure centers with people from different schools? What I experienced there gave me the idea of going back to South Texas and setting up an institute." A few years later, he won a grant from the Centers for Disease Control and Prevention (CDC) for yet another population health venture: the South Texas Border Health Disparities Center. Soon thereafter, he moved to the University of North Texas Health Science Center, where he is chair of the Department of Health Management and Policy in the School of Public Health—and where, he suspects, "I'm more attuned to interdisciplinary work than someone else might have been."

Pagán's case notwithstanding, the experience of interdisciplinary population health research, and the possibilities it opens up, do not always lead to academic careers. David Van Sickle, a medical anthropologist who was then an officer in the Epidemic Intelligence Service at the CDC, was selected in the fourth class of Health & Society Scholars, from 2006 to 2008, and at the University of Wisconsin–Madison he continued a career-long interest in asthma research. Although that research had begun in academia (his dissertation on asthma and allergy in India had been funded by the National Science Foundation), Van Sickle says, "I always knew I wasn't going to be an academic anthropologist."

Yet he was a strong candidate for the Health & Society Scholarship and a more than usually successful researcher, both during and after his stay at Wisconsin. In his work at the CDC, Van Sickle had become frustrated with the slow, fragmentary, and partial data with which epidemiologists normally have to tackle disease outbreaks. "Public health for asthma was focused on just a tiny fraction of data: hospital data and fatalities," he says. "There's information out there that could be identifying incidents, telling us key things like among whom and where, in a timely way. But at CDC we were waiting around on data sets that are years old, and then when they arrived, they'd tell us only about one percent of the events. We were never going to get very far that way. We would always be behind."

For someone with Van Sickle's career ambitions, the University of Wisconsin–Madison was an excellent fit, given that the program's leaders there welcomed scholars interested in applying their research. Not only that, but in one of his earliest experiences on campus, Van Sickle found evidence of a practical need that had already been troubling him. He recalls:

> When I got there, I realized that doctors and patients at the School of Medicine were working with the same scarcity of data that I had found so frustrating at the CDC. Even though patients are being taught to manage the disease, and docs were working in the community dealing directly with patients, none of that actual experience was being used to course-correct treatment. Docs were relying on patients to recall accurately how they'd been doing in the last three to four months since they'd last seen them. And that information wasn't all reliable. Plus, it was too episodic and dated to be very useful in the day-to-day management of the disease. Well, you could solve both problems by capturing the information on where and when asthma was affecting people in real time. You could help get doctors and communities to coordinate and do a better job working together.

Asthma is a disease with many triggers, often invisible or hard to detect. But knowing where and when patients tend to experience attacks can help doctors in guiding their patients' management of the disease, as well as in helping community health officials detect and defuse previously unknown triggers and hot spots. So in his years at Madison, Van Sickle worked with graduate students in biomedical engineering to develop a device with a global positioning system that easily attaches to most inhalers. It can instantly report to a data-tracking service the exact time and location when a patient uses the inhaler. The service, called Asthmapolis, was prototyped and tested during the scholarship period and is now part of a new start-up company led by Van Sickle and three business partners. The company has been profiled in—among many other places—a recent book titled *The Coolest Startups in America*.[5]

Although Health & Society Scholars was not designed to lead people away from university research, Van Sickle's career path is still squarely within the overall purpose of the program: to promote expansive, interdisciplinary research, thinking, and creativity in addressing the health of large populations. Although he is not likely to resume an academic career, Van Sickle and his company are tackling both practical and intellectual obstacles in society's response to disease. "Public health lags other sectors of the economy and academia in its ability to deal with data streams," he points out. "It's not now designed to make sense of a dataflow coming in in real time the way a credit card company would be, or the traffic arm of a municipality." More to the point, the solutions his research has developed are testaments to the need for multidisciplinary cooperation and teamwork in the field. They would not have been available to any one of the constituent disciplines—public health, anthropology, engineering, or advanced data management—by themselves.

And that, says Van Sickle, is largely attributable to the influence of the Health & Society scholarship. "When you first get into the program, when you spec out what you want to do and who you want to work with—that's where I first had the idea. I then vetted it with some other members of my cohort and with people at the university. That was the whole gestation of it. I knew that I wasn't going to be an anthropologist. But I wasn't at all clear about what I *was* going to do, and how I could survive while doing it. In a lot of ways, the program gave me the freedom to figure out what the path was going to look like, and to start making it happen."

The recession of 2007–2008 and the accompanying financial crash forced cutbacks in many Robert Wood Johnson Foundation programs, including Health & Society Scholars. As a result, research and training grants have been reduced along with the number of scholars, and other restraints may be needed as well. Faculty and alumni of the program have reacted to these reductions with a mixture of regret over the cuts and relief that the program will continue at a still-significant scale. As one person familiar with Health & Society Scholars put it, preferring to speak anonymously: "If the goal here were just to help some promising people do good research, it wouldn't matter much whether you supported eighteen or ten or five. But the goal is also to change the environment, the way population health research is pursued and organized and supported in the academy. That's not something you do with a handful of people on a couple of campuses. If you want real systemic change, as in any field, you have to intervene in many places for many, many years. I would hope that's still the commitment here, and I believe that it is."

—⁓— The Young Epidemiology Scholars

By aiming at relatively recent arrivals in the academic marketplace, some of whom had not yet decided on a firm career path or were willing to step off the traditional career escalator for a time, the Health & Society Scholars program sought to broaden recipients' ideas about the kind of role they could play in population health. In that respect, it hoped to have an earlier or more fundamental effect on recipients' career plans than was true in many other fellowship programs. Yet the Foundation's next step in the effort to influence careers and draw gifted people into population health would seek an even more profound influence. It would focus on an even younger generation: high school students hearing the word *epidemiology*, in many cases, for the first time. "I literally didn't know how to pronounce it," said 2010 second-place winner Jessica Hart, an aspiring harpist—and now also a public health major—from Sandy, Utah. "I had no idea what it was."

Young Epidemiology Scholars—YES for short—was inspired by the two best-known science competitions for American teenagers: the Intel Science Talent Search and the Siemens Competition. Both of these programs aim to attract and encourage the brightest young people to pursue careers in science and technology and, by publicizing the competition and the winners, to cultivate interest in these fields among other young people. Substitute "epidemiology" (or "the basic science behind population health") for "science and technology" in that description, and the result is a fairly accurate summary of YES's principal goals.

"There just wasn't a lot of excitement about a career path in public health," says senior program officer Pamela Russo, recapping the Foundation's thinking at the time the program was conceived. "Young people, when they showed some ability in math and science, were tending to go into medical school or the science labs, or maybe the social sciences. Public health wasn't getting the best and the brightest in the numbers that were going to be needed." The other science prizes seemed to be helping to generate buzz around careers in physics, chemistry, and biology, demonstrating ways that these disciplines could solve real problems and contribute to a fulfilling life. "So it was natural to think that if we're interested in developing the seed corn of the future leadership for population health," says the former senior vice president McGinnis, "then we need to have an analogue to the other scientific prize programs in the field of epidemiology."

The field's relative lack of cachet seemed integrally linked to the reaction of students like Jessica Hart: most had never heard of epidemiology or population health and had little idea what possibilities and challenges these fields might offer. To the extent that students (or, more likely, their parents) were acquainted with epidemiology or public health, their ideas were probably bound up with the outdated, disease-centric image of technicians tracking contagions or inspectors patrolling restaurant kitchens. The first purpose of Young Epidemiology Scholars was to introduce young people to the ways that the science of population health could be applied to making their communities healthier, safer, and better places to live.

As McGinnis saw it, the shortage of talent in the field could not be solved solely by supporting the smartest graduate students or newly minted PhDs. The challenge was to attract exceptional minds into the field at an early age—before they had already started traveling down some other career path. That would mean recruiting talented young people at a critical moment in their thinking about their place in the world. And it would involve stimulating their thoughts about what they could *do* in population health, what kind of difference they could make, and why it would be exciting and important.

YES began in 2003 with those goals, and it continued for eight rounds, through 2011. It was open to any high school junior or senior who wanted to develop a project in epidemiology and submit a written report on it for the national competition. Out of more than 500 competitors each year, 120 semifinalists were selected to receive at least $1,000. From that number, half progressed to the regional finals and were invited, at the program's expense, to present their projects at a two-day national event in Washington, D.C. There, the students not only gained experience presenting their research to distinguished judges, but they met and spent informal time with their fellow finalists, the judges, and other invited dignitaries. Of the 60 regional finalists, 48 students annually received $2,000 scholarships. The remaining 12 went on to present their projects one last time, before the whole assembly. Of these, 6 became national finalists and received $15,000 scholarships; two third-place winners received $20,000; two in second place won $35,000; and the top two winners each year received $50,000 apiece.

Nearly five thousand students, from every U.S. state and the District of Columbia, Puerto Rico, and American Samoa participated in the eight rounds of YES. The program was managed nationally by the College Board, which is most famous for administering the SAT, but which also manages other national prizes and scholarship programs, including the Siemens Competition. Students who take the SAT or use other College Board services can sign up to receive regular information about available sources of financial aid, and can express interest in pursuing particular subject areas such as science and health. This provided one means of contacting likely participants about the opportunity to compete in YES. But the College Board also recruited students directly, through the mail and through contact with schools and teachers. It circulated posters and sought to spread the word through media coverage, including by publicizing the national winners and the regional finalists' gathering in Washington.

Successful student projects have applied the methods of epidemiology to virtually every aspect of population health. For example, Robert Levine of Lincolnshire, Illinois, studied patterns of indoor tanning among teenagers and their awareness of the health risks; he won one of the two top prizes in the 2003–2004 round. That same year, Alanna Hay of Fort Washington, Maryland, won a $15,000 prize for research on smoking and stress among pregnant women in North Carolina. Three years later, Justin Petrillo of Westfield, New Jersey, also won $15,000 for a study of personal and ambient concentrations of a particulate air pollutant, PM2.5, in Camden, New Jersey. In the 2008–2009 competition, third-place winner Joanna Kao of Iowa City, Iowa, won $20,000 with a study of the possible roles of bilirubin and breastfeeding on retinopathy among premature infants.

"The students are all passionate, analytical, and socially conscious," says Diane Tsukamaki, director of national recognition and scholarship programs at the College Board and national program director of YES. "Their interests cover a wide range. But they haven't all been in a science program or entered any competition before. For some, it's their first. So at the national event, seeing those who are deeply involved in science interacting with students interested in other fields really gives you an idea of what an educational experience this is. The students don't just learn from their projects; they learn from each other. The experience introduces them to a wider world that many of them probably had no idea existed."

Jessica Hart, the harpist from Utah, won a $35,000 scholarship in 2010 for a study linking environmental toxins to fertility problems and fetal abnormalities among families in Salt Lake County. One of the affected women was Hart's older sister. It was that personal connection, more than any interest in science or math, that led Hart to her choice of a project—that plus the availability of a large scholarship, which she hoped to use at the prestigious Eastman School of Music in Rochester, New York. "I was looking to apply to schools out East," she recalls, "which can get pretty expensive. So when my mother read an e-mail saying there was a $50,000 scholarship available for something called epidemiology, I said, 'I have no idea what this is, but if you want, I'll do it. It can't hurt.'"

Originally inspired by her sister's experience, Hart surveyed and interviewed scores of families in the contaminated area, as well as in a comparable but uncontaminated community nearby. In the process she learned many skills, including ways of asking strangers about deeply sensitive health issues. But she also learned about the use of advanced statistics for determining patterns of risks and outcomes. "I loved collecting the data and discovering that the data could *tell* me something," she says. "I always hated math. It was a subject I just did because I had to; you just do it and get it over with. But this was about people, including someone I really cared about. And the numbers were telling me something important. That was a new experience."

Two years later, Hart is in the midst of still another new experience, one she never imagined when she entered the YES competition: in addition to majoring in harp at Eastman, she has declared a dual major at the University of Rochester, in public health. As this is written, she is under consideration for a summer internship at the CDC. As for a career choice, "I could see being an orchestral harpist or working with the CDC in environmental epidemiology. I'm still excited to learn about both, and I love what I'm doing in both of them. Luckily, I won't have to decide for a while."

Shoshanna a Goldin of Allentown, Pennsylvania, a first-place winner in the same round of competition as Jessica Hart, had no similar aversion to math or science when she entered YES. She had long set her sights on medical school, and, partly by luck, she already knew perfectly well how to pronounce *epidemiology*. Her sister Aleah had been a regional YES finalist the year before, with research on why students don't get flu shots and what kinds of communication may be effective in persuading them. Shoshanna followed her sister's entry with a project of her own, in which she studied the widespread consumption of high-energy drinks among high school students and their awareness of the risks involved. It won her $50,000 toward her tuition at Wake Forest University.

Although Goldin already had a scientific and clinical turn of mind, her YES project arose not from any prior research, but from a chance personal encounter. "At the time, energy drinks were relatively new," she remembers. "Red Bull and Monster had started popping up in my school, and I was curious why. Then one morning a friend of mine walked into my first-period class with an energy drink in his hand and two in his backpack. I asked him, 'Is that for the week, or just today?' And he said, 'No! This is just to get me through the morning!' I just stared at him."

Her resulting report, "Energy Epidemic: Teen Perceptions and Consumption of Energy Drinks," drew attention from public health officials and researchers around the country, who had only recently started documenting the effects of energy drinks on college students and adults, but had not yet focused on teens. The project not only contributed valuable new information to the field, it set in motion ripples of other activity, both in academia and public policy.

Yet for all the recognition the project and prize has won her, Goldin says that the most life-altering aspect of her YES experience was not the project itself, but "the national gathering which brings together so many distinguished people, the speakers and judges, who spend real time with us, people we would otherwise probably never have an opportunity to meet. And we learn from each other, not just seeing everyone's projects, but the relationships that form there. The scholars stay in touch after it's over, through Skype and texting and Facebook."

"These were some of the most amazing students in each academic year," she adds. "They researched a project that meant something to them and that could mean a lot to the world. That's the great thing about YES: It draws all kinds of skills and backgrounds; it's about bringing together all your skills and developing a project that really speaks to who you are and what you have to offer the community and the world."

According to James Marks, who succeeded McGinnis as Foundation senior vice president and director of the Health Group, the idea of linking one's own interests and environment with an opportunity to do something important on a large scale is what made the program work. Its appeal to students, he says, was that it

> taps into their altruism and idealism, as much as whatever interest in science they might have. They may have some familiarity with chemistry or biology, but if they do, it's probably just in laboratories. And they don't necessarily want to work on health and well-being only in laboratories. This allows them to learn the methods of scientific inquiry and population health in ways that are immersed in the difficulties of our society, of the communities where they live, and of vulnerable populations. This says to them: You can be a scientist working with people in your community, your parents with asthma, your grandparents with heart disease. You can ask, "How could I affect this? What in my community might have led to this?"

Directing would-be scholars down this path—or at least exposing them to the possibilities that might lie there—seemed a useful way of expanding the pool of talent to draw from. But the problem with that line of reasoning was that by casting such a wide net at such an early stage in life, the Foundation could have no way of being sure that it was reaching the right people with the right kind of intervention. Some scholarship recipients might well have chosen a population health career anyway, award or no. Others might benefit from the award, learn a great deal from participating, but then pursue different careers entirely. Career decisions at age eighteen tend to change, often profoundly, by age twenty-five. Especially among very bright students, many opportunities will open unexpectedly along the route to adulthood. So it is difficult, maybe impossible, to know how much one experience, no matter how rich and rewarding, could influence choices made four, eight, or fifteen years later.

Those kinds of uncertainties, which had been raised from time to time since the earliest years of the program, ultimately helped bring it to a close. The demands of fiscal restraint in a harsh economy added to the pressure on YES, as did the awkward fit between a program aimed at teenagers and a foundation whose other fellowships mainly support postdoctoral and midcareer research. Any one of these concerns—shrinking budgets, strategic misalignment, or quandaries over impact and measurement—might have been overlooked in the interest of experimenting with an intriguing (and, many people added, inspiring) new kind of scholarship. But all three together were more than the program could withstand.

Yet many of the people who observed YES most closely remain convinced that it filled an important gap in philanthropy's effort to draw the brightest young minds into population health. David Van Sickle, the Health & Society Scholar, also served as a judge in every round of the YES competition except the last. He argues that the issue of career choices is less important than the opportunity the program offered to steep young people in

the fundamental skills of epidemiology, like methods of inquiry, critical thinking, hypothesis generation, quantitative analysis. Our economy needs—and society needs—more people who understand these basic approaches and methods. Some will use them in epidemiology; some will use them in other fields. But *more* will use them in epidemiology and public health if we expose them early and inspire them. And in any case, public health isn't just something professionals do; you get better public health when you have a more thoughtful public. So to me, a focus on high school students was really smart. Maybe this was not the place for it; maybe there are other ways to do it. But the value of it I think is beyond question.

~~~ Conclusion: Thoughts on Building a Field from the Bottom Up

Whether aiming at teenagers or early-career researchers, the two fellowship programs described here have sought to recruit early, embryonic talent into a broadly defined field that the Foundation considered generally underpopulated. In the past, most Robert Wood Johnson Foundation programs for scholars aimed at accomplished people already on a specified professional track. The touchstone Clinical Scholars program, for example, is limited to physicians. The Health Policy Fellowships are awarded to health professionals who have completed residencies and are thus steeped in their specialty areas. Later programs, such as Scholars in Health Policy Research, did seek out more junior recipients. But these programs generally helped scholars excel on more traditionally defined career paths to which they were already committed—though many shifted their emphasis to health: for example, from labor economics to health economics. There have been occasional exceptions, to be sure—particularly programs to attract more minority students into medicine and nursing. But these, too, were relatively specific as to the kinds of careers they hoped to inspire young people to join.

By contrast, although Health & Society Scholars and YES clearly hoped to point their recipients toward a commitment to population health, they accepted a high degree of risk that this hope might be disappointed. They actively sought out gifted young people whose career paths were either partly or, in the case of YES, completely unmapped. It is probably significant that this approach took shape at about the same time that the Foundation was seeking to invest more in health, to balance its support for more traditional health care. Population health is still a loosely defined field whose future depends on recruiting talent from many branches of the natural and social sciences and the humanities. Consequently, to many people at the Foundation, moving a step or two away from narrowly targeted fellowships and toward programs with more open, permissive eligibility criteria seemed natural—even necessary.

As the former senior vice president J. Michael McGinnis recalls it, particularly in designing Health & Society Scholars, "We borrowed quite specifically from the model of the Clinical Scholars program, attracting the best and brightest and funding centers of learning where they could flourish. But it was clear that we needed to move beyond clinicians; in fact we could not start with them. We had to, first, bring in people from multiple disciplines, and second, focus not just on their particular fields of expertise—whether medicine or law or economics or molecular biology—but also on the cross-cutting relationships of people working with one another across disciplines." The movement beyond individual disciplines was even more pronounced in YES, where participants would not yet have any career path at all.

It is possible, though difficult, to measure the value of these kinds of early-career fellowships. A rigorous evaluation, such as a randomized controlled trial, would be prohibitively difficult if not impossible; yet as evaluations of Clinical Scholars and Scholars in Health Policy Research have shown, there are ways to judge the general effectiveness of investments in individuals, even when the evidence is visible only many years later. David Colby, the Foundation vice president for research and evaluation, notes that such evaluations, though lacking the certainty of a randomized experiment, can track "people's intellectual contributions, and the interactions of those contributions with other developments in the field, seeing what they write and where they get published, which publications are judged as influential or breakthrough. Given enough time—and this could mean at least ten years in the case of Health & Society Scholars, and more like twenty-five or thirty years in the case of YES—you could follow each individual, see patterns of influence and career trajectory, the grants they're getting, their leadership positions, where they're asked to speak, and so on."

Foundation fellowship programs are all eventually subjected to those kinds of evaluations, and Colby expects that the Health & Society Scholars will be evaluated in roughly this way as well. Meanwhile, the participating universities are steadily compiling many of the indicators relevant to such an evaluation: publications by scholars and alumni in peer-reviewed journals, grants received, and funded research projects under way. Yet without a firm basis of comparison or control, he acknowledges that the results will mostly involve "qualitative, expert judgment and assessment," drawing from informed observation and surmise, rather than furnishing any kind of numerical certainty. Still, such evaluations produce a sound basis for judgment and decision making, and "the best conclusions you can reasonably reach about programs that are inherently long-term and complex."

Such imponderables are endemic to the kind of philanthropy that focuses on cultivating individual talent rather than delivering services, solving specific problems, or altering markets. And admittedly, the quandaries only become greater the earlier one tries to intervene in the careers of talented young people. Yet for all the uncertainties, investment in "human capital"—even at very early stages—is probably the world's oldest and most revered form of philanthropy, as popular now as it was in imperial Rome or Renaissance Florence. (When the Medici supported a fifteen-year-old artist's apprentice named Leonardo, they had no idea the world would end up with the *Mona Lisa*, but they must have been satisfied that something good would result.) In these cases, the "expert judgment and assessment" approach has always been the best, and most often the only, root of decision making.

Harvey Fineberg, president of the Institute of Medicine and a close observer of both the Health & Society Scholars program—he is chair of its advisory committee—and YES, says, "We need more of this kind of philanthropy, not less. And by 'we,' I mean society. These kinds of programs add a great deal to the life opportunities, knowledge, and experience of people who in turn are going to add a great deal to society's well-being. If you can't say with certainty exactly how much it adds, you can certainly conclude that it makes a difference. I personally think if you quadrupled it, it would not saturate the need or the market. It's a finite, attractive intervention that can reinforce and shape choices that will shape a lifetime."

Notes

1. Association of Schools of Public Health, "ASPH Policy Brief: Confronting the Public Health Workforce Crisis," December 2008, p. 4, http://www.asph.org/document.cfm?page=1038.
2. It's telling that not all population health experts believe the word "field" applies, or even should apply, to their area of work. Some instead view their domain as more of a crossroads where other fields come together. This partly semantic debate is beyond the scope of this article, except to point out that even those who disavow the term "field" still generally hope to build the key assets listed here: communication networks, centers of collaboration, and routinely interdisciplinary modes and standards of practice.
3. Isaacs, S. L., Sandy, L. G., and Schroeder, S. A. "Improving the Health Care Workforce: Perspectives from Twenty-Four Years' Experience." *To Improve Health and Health Care 1997: The Robert Wood Johnson Foundation Anthology*. San Francisco: Jossey-Bass, p. 13, http://rwjf.org/files /research/anthology97chapter2.pdf.
4. Grant amounts have varied over the years; amounts given here are for 2012.
5. Bloch, D. *The Coolest Startups in America (Volume 1)*. New York: Building Bloch Books, 2012.

CHAPTER 12

Child FIRST: A Program to Help Very Young At-Risk Children

Digby Diehl

Editors' Introduction

Although never formally denoted a Robert Wood Johnson Foundation priority, improving children's health has occupied an important place in the Foundation's grantmaking.[1] Since 1972, the Foundation has allocated more than $2 billion to programs aimed at making children healthier. Many of them have focused on improving the health of infants and young children. Back in 1975, the Foundation launched the Regionalized Perinatal Care Program, which organized hospitals in eight areas of the country into regional networks to make perinatal technology available to more women and their at-risk babies. This led to the Rural Infant Care Program in 1979, which expanded perinatal networks to some of the country's most isolated communities. It was followed, beginning in 1982, by the largest, at the time, randomized control trial on infants' health undertaken in the United States. The Nurse Home Visitation program (now known as the Nurse-Family Partnership program), under which nurses visit poor, pregnant women in their homes and counsel them for two years after the baby's birth, is one of the Foundation's signature efforts and stands as a well-documented evidence-based intervention.

Firmly rooted in this history is Child FIRST, a family-based intervention that focuses on preventing mental health problems in high-risk mothers and young children. The brainchild of a dynamic pediatrician named Darcy Lowell, Child FIRST was initially funded by the Foundation through its Local Initiative Funding Partners program (now known as the Robert Wood Johnson Foundation Local Funding Partnerships program). Child FIRST has shown promising results in Bridgeport, Connecticut, and is now being replicated throughout the state and beyond. Despite the difficult economic times, which can threaten the viability of resource-intensive programs such as Child FIRST, the State of Connecticut allocated funds to expand the program.

In this chapter, Digby Diehl, a writer whose most recent book, *Rather Outspoken*, a collaboration with Dan Rather, appeared earlier this year, discusses this innovative program and its replication.

"Come and get your child!" the mother was told. "He hits and bites other children. He throws toys. He kicks the teachers. He screams and cries constantly. We are expelling your son from preschool. As of now."

This was the third school the little boy had attended in less than a year. He'd been a happy three-year-old until the FBI arrived at his home in the middle of the night, lights flashing, sirens blaring. They busted down the door, pushed his mother to the floor, and dragged his father away in handcuffs.

After the father was convicted of drug trafficking, the mother became depressed, but still took her son to visit his father in the high-security prison where he was incarcerated. The setting was so frightening that the boy vomited repeatedly every time he went. Shunned by her own family, the mother spiraled into deep depression. She stopped bathing; she stopped getting dressed. She sat in the darkened apartment all day long. The traumatized boy began showing symptoms of abandonment and rejection. His behavior at preschool was his way of lashing out in rage and confusion at what was happening to his family.

—⁓— "Behavior Is Meaningful Communication"

What is going on when a very young child's behavior is so disruptive that he or she gets expelled from preschool or day care? What's happening in that child's life that might cause this to happen? Too often, these questions are not being asked.

But they are precisely the questions that Child FIRST asks. Child FIRST is a Connecticut-based intensive, early childhood home-visiting intervention program that works with the state's most vulnerable young children (up to age six) and their families. Its goal is to "identify young children and families with serious challenges and provide comprehensive assessment, parent–child intervention, and connection to broad, well integrated services and supports in order to prevent serious emotional disturbance, developmental and learning problems, and abuse and neglect." Originally based in Bridgeport, the Child FIRST program has expanded to New Haven, Norwalk, Hartford, Waterbury, and New London, and will soon be available throughout Connecticut.

"Behavior is meaningful communication," says pediatrician Darcy Lowell, the founder and executive director of Child FIRST. "Everything a child does has meaning. In very young children, what we have come to call 'acting out' is a really a cry for help." Lowell continues, "We know that in very young children, serious emotional and psychological problems, developmental delays, and learning disabilities are often linked to family stress due to poverty and violence. Nevertheless, these issues are commonly overlooked in the rush to simply 'fix' the child's troublesome behavior and make it go away. At Child FIRST, we do not just respond to a behavior. We identify and respond to the underlying factors that are generating it."

To do so, Child FIRST works with children and parents in their homes, using a two-pronged approach. One prong fosters a closer and more stable emotional relationship between parent and child. The other is designed to dial down the level of environmental stress by dealing with the family's concrete needs for basic necessities. Each prong reinforces the other as a clinician and a care coordinator work in tandem to deliver the program. Both must have experience working with young children and their families and have been educated in a field such as social work, family therapy, psychiatric nursing, or psychology—clinicians at the master's degree level, care coordinators at the bachelor's degree level. In Child FIRST terms, they "wrap around" the family to address their problems, both large and small.

—∿— The Beginnings of Child FIRST

Darcy Lowell has been interested in child health and well-being since her own childhood. "Growing up, I always knew I was going to be involved with children," she says. "When I was in college,

I became interested in the psychiatric and psychological problems of young children. In medical school I switched to pediatrics, because the pediatricians saw children when they were babies. Psychiatrists rarely saw children before they were five or six years old."

A summa cum laude graduate of Yale University, Lowell was in its first class of women. She describes herself as a bulldog—and not just because it is the Yale mascot. Lowell is both passionate and tenacious about helping young children, and credits her upbringing with her choice to work with vulnerable and at-risk children and their families. "My father was a lawyer and my mother was a social worker," she says. "Both were very interested in social justice issues. My father was deputy mayor of New York under Robert Wagner, and then in 1960 became the first chairman of the city's Commission on Human Rights. My mother gave me great insight into the people side of things—she cared a lot about the families she worked with, especially the children. My parents also encouraged me to believe that I could make things better if I put my mind to it. If I thought something was important and I put my energy into it, I could make it happen. That was the culture I grew up in, and it became part of me—it's in my blood."

As a young pediatrician, Lowell became a fellow in a Robert Wood Johnson Foundation program at Yale. "This was a General Academic Pediatrics program that was an appealing combination of a research fellowship, a teaching fellowship, and a clinical fellowship. Eventually I took a position at Bridgeport Hospital, where in 1986 I became the director of the Child Development Clinic and Consultation Service. This job gave me some much-needed flexibility, since by this time I was a new mother, and I understood the importance of spending time with my child. I ran the child development clinic in the hospital, and did one-on-one consultations with local Bridgeport community service providers."

By this time, Bridgeport was already a city in decline. For more than a century, it had been a prosperous industrial town—circus showman P. T. Barnum is the city's most famous resident, and was for a time its mayor. One of Bridgeport's early industries was the Frisbie Pie Company, whose disc-shaped pie tins gave rise to the toy we know as the Frisbee. Beginning in the 1970s, however, Bridgeport's manufacturing base started to erode, and the city began a protracted economic skid.

It has yet to really recover. With a population of just under 145,000 people, Bridgeport is still the most populous city in Connecticut. Although larger than either Hartford or New Haven, today Bridgeport's most dubious distinction is that according to 2010 census data, it is the center of a metropolitan area with the most unequal income distribution in America.[2] In the Bridgeport-Stamford-Norwalk metropolitan area, the richest 5 percent of the population earns $49 for each $1 earned by the poorest 5 percent. Approximately 23 percent of all Bridgeport families fall below the poverty line, nearly double the state average. Even worse, more than 30 percent of Bridgeport's children live in poverty, compared with a state average of 12 percent.

In her role as director of the child development clinic at Bridgeport Hospital, Lowell dealt on a daily basis with the devastating effects that this harsh economic climate was creating for the city's poorest children. "I was seeing lots of young children with developmental delays. Back then, children who were behind in language development were given speech and language therapy, but no one was asking why they were behind," she recalls. "These children came from families with multiple challenges in their lives. They were victims of poverty. They had insufficient access to health care, nutrition, and decent housing. Beyond that, no one was looking into the broader issues these families were coping with—domestic violence, substance abuse, homelessness, mental illness."

Because she was still consulting individually with a variety of local educational and social services agencies, Lowell saw an opportunity to forge the missing connection. "I was dealing with people from many different organizations that were all working on aspects of the same problem," she says, "but no one was connecting the dots and looking at the larger picture. I knew that we couldn't just look at the child in isolation. It was essential to consider the child in the constellation of everything going on in his or her world."

At Lowell's instigation, some of the providers she'd been consulting with started meeting informally to discuss the problem. "In the beginning, we had people from the schools, from early care and education, a neurologist, someone from the health department … It was a very open group. If you wanted to join us, you were invited. We met weekly, because there were so many children who needed help. Everyone brought their thorniest, most difficult cases to our meetings—these were children and families that had fallen through the cracks."

In the early 1990s, the kind of interagency effort Lowell put together was uncommon, but in their face-to-face meetings it became clear that each of the participants held a piece of the solution. The group realized that they needed to pool their resources and expertise to put together a case-specific strategy that dealt not only with the problems of the child, but also with the problems of the family.

They began working to fit the pieces together. Within this collaborative environment, individuals and agency representatives stepped up and volunteered to take on whatever piece of the problem was within their purview. The result was an integrated, comprehensive plan for each case. It proved to be effective, even where prior efforts had failed. "With providers coming together for a systems approach, issues of turf dissolved," says Lowell. "Our task force began as an ad hoc collaborating problem-solving group. We called it 'The First Team,' but it was really the genesis of Child FIRST."

"Darcy Lowell's approach was collaborative from day one," says June Malone, who participated in the meetings as a representative of Action for Bridgeport Community Development (ABCD), which encompasses Bridgeport's Head Start program. "Bridgeport was seeing increasing numbers of children expelled from child care and preschool for behavioral problems that teachers and daycare providers just couldn't deal with. Even before the formal establishment of Child FIRST, Darcy brought together representatives from many agencies in Bridgeport that had an interest in child welfare, child development, and early childhood education. As service providers and stakeholders, we identified areas that needed to be addressed as a community, and how we could work in partnership."

The collaborative officially became Child FIRST in 2001. The "FIRST" in Child FIRST is actually an acronym, standing for Family, Interagency, Resource, Support, and Training, and reflects the program's ongoing comprehensive, collaborative, and interdisciplinary approach. That same year, Lowell received a grant from the Connecticut Health Foundation to create an "early childhood mental health system of care" for the Bridgeport area.

—⚬⚬— The Child FIRST Model: A System of Care

The Child FIRST program that evolved from those early efforts has both community and home intervention components.

- Screening/Early Identification/Referrals
- Work with Schools and Preschools
- Home Intervention
  - Comprehensive Assessment of Child and Family Needs
  - Development of a Child and Family Plan of Care
  - Care Coordination/Case Management
  - Parent–Child Mental Health Intervention

Screening/Early Identification/Referrals

Children and families are referred to Child FIRST through a variety of avenues, including pediatricians, neighbors, relatives, schools, and preschools. Because those who need help the most can be the hardest to find, Child FIRST also casts a wide net, making outreach efforts to high-risk families through homeless shelters; adult mental health, substance abuse, and domestic violence programs; the courts; and the Connecticut Department of Children and Families.

Supported by a Robert Wood Johnson Foundation grant, in 2006 Child FIRST Bridgeport started screening children for emotional and behavioral problems and environmental risks. Screening took place both in local preschools and at the pediatric clinic in the Bridgeport Hospital Primary Care Center. Almost half—47 percent—screened positive for emotional behavioral problems, and 40 percent tested positive for social/environmental risk. Although the hospital screening program remains in place, for doctors and nurses the first indication of a problem often comes from basic observation—looking at the way parents and children interact, or perhaps do not interact. "We might see a child who is very out of control in the examining room, and a mom not even trying to control him," says Allyson Driggers, the clinic's medical director. "That makes my antennae go up. If I ask the mom what's going on, she might say, 'Oh, this kid is really horrible. He never listens.' The next question I ask is, 'How do you handle that situation?'"

Not surprisingly, the mother's answer often helps to pinpoint the problem. "We have many teenage moms who don't have good parenting skills because they were not well parented themselves," explains Driggers. "We refer families to Child FIRST so they can help moms learn a better way to interact with their children. We reap the benefits of the services they provide for our patients, and our families don't wind up dealing with DCF."

The DCF is a state agency, Connecticut's Department of Children and Families, and for many parents the prospect of DCF involvement is seen as a grave threat because it has the legal authority to go to court to remove a child from the home.

Through DCF, Child FIRST began working with three-year-old twin brothers. For their safety and well-being, DCF had taken them from their parents when they were just six months old. By the time they were three, the twins had already been in two foster homes. Both boys exhibited behavioral difficulties, so neither of the foster placements worked out. After a single mom—a schoolteacher—offered to adopt the boys, Child FIRST was called in to work with her. "We are supporting her in the process of learning how to care for these challenging boys," says Norka Malberg, a psychotherapist who serves as clinical director at Child FIRST. "It is difficult, but this mother is extremely reflective. She's strong and has a good social-support network. Our work is to help her advocate for what she needs in terms of being a single mother of twin boys with a traumatic past. We are helping her find the right classroom for them, and helping teachers understand their needs."

Although these boys were removed as infants from their birth home because both parents were mentally ill, the Department of Children and Families is increasingly reluctant to take this action, except as a last resort. "DCF is moving away from what had been a punitive role—you're a bad mother and we are going to take your child away—and toward trying to lend families a helping hand," says Maria Brereton, DCF's Regional Administrator for Region I (Bridgeport).

Helping parents do better with their children so the family can stay together is one of the primary reasons DCF refers families to Child FIRST. "Research tells us that children do better if they stay with their families in a home environment," Brereton continues. "I jumped into the deep end with Darcy Lowell and formalized a contract with Child FIRST because they help families avoid having their problems escalate to the point where they need state intervention."

Brereton talks about the case of a young boy with developmental problems:

> He was placed in a group home because his parents didn't know how to take care of him. He'd been there for about a year. Several of our child welfare staff professionals were recommending that we terminate parental rights, because the mom and dad had been unable

to keep him safe. I asked whether the parents were still visiting their son. They were, like clockwork. That's when I asked Child FIRST to get involved. They worked with the parents to improve their parenting skills, and they were able to bring their son home. If we had terminated their parental rights, this little boy would have been placed with total strangers at the age of six. That often is a set-up for lifelong repercussions. There was an excellent chance that I'd be dealing with this boy again in ten years, when he was getting arrested, or getting referred to a psychiatric hospital.

Work with Schools and Preschools

Child FIRST clinicians teach skills and strategies to teachers who have at-risk children in their classrooms. In Bridgeport, Child FIRST began providing classroom and mental health coaching in preschools in 2003. "I was in the classroom doing observation and I saw children who were very clearly playing out something traumatic that had happened at home," says ABCD Head Start's June Malone. "I knew their play had a serious root cause, and I knew we needed to give our teachers more skills. We asked Child FIRST to help teachers understand the meaning of difficult behaviors, and to coach them on how to deal with it. After that, we saw wonderful gains in our staff skills. We not only stopped kicking kids out for behavior, we also had our teachers volunteering to take the children other teachers wanted to get rid of. We got referral calls from the Board of Education and DCF saying, 'We've got a kid who has failed in three other programs,' and we'd say, 'Send him here.'"

Child FIRST clinicians also work with schools and preschools as part of a family home-intervention program (discussed in the following section). For a preschool child, the clinician will meet with teachers and observe the child in the educational setting. As the clinician comes to a fuller understanding of the problems triggering the child's behavior, he or she works with the teaching staff to find a way to enhance and reinforce the child's social and emotional development.

The collaboration works in the opposite direction as well—if a school or preschool has a child who is exhibiting disturbing behaviors, it may ask Child FIRST to get involved with the family. One family was referred to Child FIRST after their son had started flipping over desks in preschool. He was also being aggressive with other children. "Like so many of our little guys and girls, he had experienced some things in his life that were hard for him to understand," says Christine Montgomery, who administers the Child FIRST program at Clifford W. Beers Guidance Clinic in New Haven. "He had witnessed some pretty significant violence between his mom and dad, and his dad had a history of being incarcerated. It was not too hard to track it back."

Home Intervention

Child FIRST tailors its approach to meet the specific needs of each child and family, but in developing that individualized program, clinicians build on the basic components of the Child FIRST model. These components are described in the following sections.

Comprehensive Assessment of Child and Family Needs

After a referral has been made, Child FIRST clinicians and care coordinators must establish a relationship with the family. Once the door opens, the clinician focuses on the family's emotional needs, in particular on the relationship between the parent and the child. The care coordinator focuses on the physical needs of the family—for families facing immediate crisis, this is frequently the beginning point. "We meet the family where it's at," says Child FIRST clinical director Malberg. "Heat, light, beds, pest control, winter clothing, diapers, shoes ... we make every effort to help our families obtain these basic items. This effort reinforces the idea that we are attentive to their needs, and that we are reliable. It reassures them that we are on their side."

"Going into people's homes gives us a chance to see what their lives are really like. There could be chaos. There might be strangers coming and going to whom you are not introduced. There could be five children screaming in the other room. It's important never to judge," Lowell says. She continues:

> I remember going into one house. It was dark. The shades were all ripped, and they were pulled all the way down. The floors were wood, but all around the edges there were sharp tacks that at one time had held a rug in place—sharp edges that would hurt a child. There were broken tiles in the bathroom—more sharp edges. The paint was peeling and there were cockroaches everywhere. This family was obviously living under very difficult circumstances. Yes, there were conditions in the home that were dangerous to small children, but we have to help families, not judge them. We work from the understanding that people are doing the best they can—that they want to be good parents. They just don't know how.

Patience and persistence are essential. Silvia Juarez, the clinician who worked with the little boy at the beginning of this story, slipped notes under the door of the boy's home every day for six weeks before his mother would let her in. Even then, the mom was wary. Winning the family's trust and confidence can become even more challenging once parents realize that the Child FIRST program goes beyond "fixing" the behavioral problems of their son or daughter.

Early on, the Child FIRST team works with the family to complete a detailed written assessment of the family's needs and psychosocial history. "It's part of the engagement process," says Bridgeport clinician Donna Vitulano. "We have a lot of measures that we have families complete—on developmental and behavioral needs, parental mood, as well psychosocial stressors in the home and in the community."

"We need to make sure that the family understands why we're here," says Adriana Lorduy, the care coordinator who is the other half of Donna Vitulano's team. "We tell families in advance about the assessment, what it's for, and how the information is going to be used to help them."

Once they understand that the assessment will benefit them, most parents cooperate. Some, however, bristle at the intrusion and are troubled by the idea of divulging so much personal information. "Sometimes we can't do the assessments right away, because there's too much stuff going on," says care coordinator Alicia Cruz. "Parents shut down. If it's too heavy in the home, even taking out a piece of paper can be intimidating. If we start working on the assessment forms before we have really established a relationship of trust, they'll send us right out the door."

The team jumps through almost any hoop to create that relationship of trust, and to demonstrate that they are on the side of the family. Assessment occurs primarily in the home, but initial meetings may take place in almost any venue where the family is comfortable. "We meet them wherever and whenever they prefer," says Lowell. "If they miss an appointment, we'll schedule another one."

Development of a Child and Family Plan of Care

Child FIRST develops the plan not *for* the family, but *with* the family. "It is essential that we remain respectful of the family's wishes and desires, and of their culture," says Lowell. "Change grows out of a relationship of trust—between parent and child, and between parents and Child FIRST. The way we deal with parents helps them understand how to have a different relationship with their children. It's all about relationships."

"When families begin working with us, they often don't know exactly what they're in for," says Child FIRST clinical supervisor Christine Montgomery. "We work a lot with the term 'family vision': Where do you want your family to be, and how can we help you get there?" For many families, it's the first time anyone has asked them that question. "We talk with families about their faith and their culture and their extended family," she continues. "We do a lot of building on the family's natural supports, because those are the underpinnings that are going to sustain them after we're gone."

The plan of care includes not only services for the child, but also services and supports for parents and siblings. Once in place, the plan is reviewed every three months, or more often if the family situation changes.

Care Coordination/Case Management

The role of the care coordinator is to help the family gain access to services and assistance. Care coordinators must have community-specific knowledge about resources they can tap into to assist the family with basic needs such as food, clothing, and housing. They must also know how to access health care services for issues such as domestic violence, substance abuse, and maternal depression.

The recent economic downturn and subsequent governmental belt-tightening has made this facet of the Child FIRST program more important but also more challenging. Some families have difficulty getting access to food stamps or federal WIC (Women, Infants and Children) food packages, even if they have been eligible for them before. And this past winter, Connecticut cut back significantly on the amount of money allocated for heating assistance for poor families.

Often lost in what can be a maze of bureaucratic red tape, families who are most in need can be denied services and benefits to which they are entitled—because of their inability to work the system. The care coordinator helps parents fill out forms and serves as a liaison with government agencies. As work with the family continues, the care coordinator teaches the parents how to access services on their own.

It is not uncommon for Child FIRST to enter the scene when the lack of basic necessities is already acute. "Often the first priority is to address the unmet urgent needs," says Alice Forrester, executive director of the Clifford W. Beers Guidance

Clinic, Child FIRST's lead agency in New Haven. "Is there heat? Is there food in the home? Is there a home? Is the family about to lose its home? We start at the crisis, and then get to the work."

Parent-Child Mental Health Intervention

"The work," as Forrester calls it, is the therapeutic component of the intervention, directed toward establishing a stronger and healthier relationship between parents and child—or more often, between the mother and her child. Although Child FIRST staff is always happy to work with fathers, the majority of cases involve single mothers.

Child FIRST teams work in the home because there they can address issues in their natural setting. In practice, this means that clinicians spend a lot of time on the floor, facilitating play between the mothers and their babies. As they watch the mom and child together, clinicians use open-ended questions to get her to reflect on the meaning of her child's behavior. "When his eyes turn away like that, what do you imagine he's thinking?" They also look for "teachable moments" to encourage the mom to see the world from her child's point of view. "What do you suppose it's like for him when we can't quite figure out what he's trying to tell us?"

The Child FIRST intervention is grounded in attachment theory, which underlies child–parent psychotherapy. Enter the "Ghosts in the Nursery." These shadowy and potentially formidable adversaries are Selma Fraiberg's personification of the phenomenon that in parenting, history tends to repeat itself, either for better or for worse.[3] Mothers raise their children in the same way they were raised—even if they had been neglected or abused when they were girls. Without help, these parents often fall into the same pattern they experienced as children, even if that pattern was traumatic or pathological.

For infants to form a secure attachment with the parent, mothers need to really connect with their children by voice, touch, and eye contact, but this may be unfamiliar to them if they never experienced it themselves. "Maybe that mom never had a cuddle as a child," says Child FIRST's Norka Malberg. "Maybe her own mother was remote or unresponsive. Maybe she suffered some sort of trauma."

The Child FIRST intervention breaks the negative cycle by guiding mothers to revisit their own histories and confront their own ghosts. With the youngest preverbal children, this often means that clinicians themselves give voice to the child's needs. "Mothers may be initially startled," says Malberg, "to hear their clinician say in a baby-like voice, 'Mommy, I'm very sad right now. I think you need to pick me up. I need a cuddle.'" Child FIRST teams help mothers understand that even preverbal children have the ability to express their needs, and that these needs are separate from those of the mother.

This may be a difficult concept to get across, especially with traumatized, inexperienced, or immature young mothers. "When we speak for the baby," says Gail Melanson, the clinical director of the Child FIRST program in Norwalk, "we do it to heighten the mom's awareness that her child, even as an infant, already has his or her own mind, his or her own capacity to take in the world around them."

Many parents who are referred to Child FIRST were themselves removed from their families when they were younger. They have a multigenerational history of involvement with Connecticut's Department of Children and Families. "We've been working with a mom who has been in the system forever," says Malberg. "As a young child, her mother died of AIDS, and she was raised by her paternal grandparents. They did the best they could, but she had a lot of difficulties as an adolescent. She became a teenage mom; she had two children by her first partner, who was a very violent man. He ended up in jail, and she lost parental rights to those two kids.

"When she was referred to us, she was only twenty years old. She had just had her third baby. The father of this child was also in jail, but not for anything violent—he owed support to his ex-wife. We started working with this mother when her child was just two weeks old. We wanted to give her the parenting tools and the help she needed so she didn't have to surrender this baby as well.

"We tried to reflect with this mom about what it meant to have this third child, a child she's hoping to keep. We went every week for an hour and a half. We sat on the floor with the mom and the baby, and we talked. When the baby's father got out of jail, we invited him into the sessions. He'd never had any contact with his child, and for a while the focus of the work was on integrating the father back into the family, helping the mother get used to having the dad in the relationship. The care coordinator helped the father find a job, and helped the family find a better home. Now this young woman, for the first time in her life, actually has the sense of having her own place, with a partner who is involved with his child and doesn't hurt her.

"The care coordinator also started working with the young mom on getting into an education program so she can get her GED," Malberg continues. "Everything was going pretty well until the father of her first two children was released from prison. This added another dimension to our work; we had to work with the parents on the importance of how to stay safe. Part of it entails thinking with the mom about her relationship with this other man, about the pattern of behavior that led her to let this man hurt her—what was there in her history of trauma that was becoming a barrier for her psychologically to be able to stand up and protect herself?"

Above all, of course, the Child FIRST team works on how to prevent the violence from happening again. If necessary, the care coordinator will encourage the mother to file for a restraining order and help her with the paperwork.

—ᴧᴧ— The Research Behind Child FIRST

The Child FIRST model is supported by recent groundbreaking research in the field of early childhood mental development, much of it by Jack Shonkoff, a pediatrician and the director of Harvard's Center on the Developing Child.[4] His research has proven conclusively that a very young child's experiences and environment profoundly influence brain growth and development, even the architecture of the brain itself.

By the age of just three years, 80 percent of brain development is complete. Infants and toddlers who are happy, sheltered, and stimulated by their environment and by contact with parents and other caregivers develop a robust web of neural networks and interconnections in the brain. In particular it is the loving, secure, playful give-and-take between parent and child that promotes the vigorous growth and expansion of this web, which serves as both springboard and scaffolding for future learning and development. Sadly, what is groundbreaking in Shonkoff's research is heartbreaking as well. Infants and toddlers who are not happy, not sheltered, and not stimulated do not develop this healthy web of interconnections. On the contrary, sustained exposure to extreme stress, often called toxic stress, produces neural networks that are stunted, frayed, truncated, or miswired.[5]

The underlying physiology behind this breakneck pace in early childhood is the remarkable capacity of the very young brain to take in almost everything around it. But brain plasticity falls off steeply after age six, and the window to effect improvement in at-risk children slams shut rapidly after that. In affection- and stimulation-deprived children, age six is when unused brain cells—cells that would have been part of a healthy neural network—begin to atrophy and die off. By the time a child is in the third or fourth grade, intervention and any needed treatment become more expensive and more prolonged. Worse yet, the chances of success begin to decline markedly, as does the degree of remediation that might be achieved. Early intervention with at-risk children—while the window is still open—is key if these permanent negative effects are to be avoided or mitigated.

~~ The Robert Wood Johnson Foundation's Initial Support of Child FIRST

In 2005, through the Local Initiative Funding Partners program (now the Local Funding Partnerships program), the Robert Wood Johnson Foundation made a four-year, $500,000 grant to Child FIRST to support its work in Bridgeport. Then as now, Child FIRST had many funding partners, including the Connecticut Department of Children and Families, The Children's Fund of Connecticut, the United Way of Eastern Fairfield County, and the Connecticut Health Foundation.

"It was clear from the grant application that the situation was horrific, not only for the children and their families, but for teachers and day-care workers as well," says Pauline Seitz, director of the Local Funding Partnerships program. "No one knew how to manage these children. Families were frustrated because they had to take the child into an institutional setting—to the child psychiatrist and the child therapist. The idea that these children could be helped more effectively in their own homes was impressive."

Anecdotal reports had strongly pointed to the effectiveness of the Child FIRST approach in improving the emotional health of very young children. To confirm the accuracy of those observations, Child FIRST had already secured funding from the federal Substance Abuse and Mental Health Services Administration (SAMHSA) to conduct a rigorous, randomized trial of their model. After the data had been collected, however, there weren't enough financial resources available to get it analyzed.

In 2007, on the recommendation of the Local Initiative Funding Partners program, the Robert Wood Johnson Foundation made a $125,000 follow-on grant to Child FIRST to complete the evaluation—as well as to conduct a cost-benefit analysis, to secure expanded Medicaid reimbursement through DCF certification as an "evidence-based program" within Connecticut, and to develop program materials and training for the model's replication.

The Evaluation of Child FIRST

Once the data was processed, trial results confirmed the positive and statistically significant outcomes for Child FIRST intervention. At the twelve-month follow-up, Child FIRST children were almost five times less likely to display aggressive or deviant behaviors, and more than four times less likely to have language problems. Mothers who had participated with Child FIRST also had significantly reduced levels of depression. The most pronounced change took place not in the first six months of working with Child FIRST, but between six and twelve months of intervention. Care coordinators helped highly stressed Child FIRST families gain three times more access to much-needed social services.[6]

Program Expansion

In 2009, the Robert Wood Johnson Foundation awarded $3.2 million to Child FIRST to expand into four additional regions of Connecticut: New Haven, Hartford, Norwalk, and Waterbury. Expansion at each site worked through a local lead agency: Clifford W. Beers Guidance Clinic in New Haven, the Village for Families & Children in Hartford, the Child Guidance Center of Mid-Fairfield County in Norwalk, and Wellpath in Waterbury. All sites were up and running by April 2010. An additional Child FIRST venue at New London was funded by SAMHSA, making a total of six Child FIRST sites.

Beyond adding these new sites, however, the grant was used to prepare the groundwork for further expansion. There were eight primary goals of the grant:

- Establish an interagency state-level executive committee to oversee the development and implementation of the initiative.

- Select four Connecticut cities as replication sites, including Hartford and New Haven.

- Establish the Replication Coordination Center to provide intensive training and ensure fidelity to key elements of the model.

- Obtain certification for Medicaid reimbursement for diagnosed children at all Child FIRST sites and advocate for increased reimbursement rates.

- Advocate for the expansion of Medicaid reimbursement to cover preventive services, before a child shows significant symptoms.

- Develop a web-based data system to manage data on process and outcomes across all sites.

- Analyze outcomes data to document effectiveness and disseminate results, including publication in a national peer-reviewed journal.

- Apply to the federal government for certification as an evidence-based model.

- Engage funding partners in a public-private partnership to support replication of Child FIRST and integration of the model with the state's early childhood system of services.

Replication—with fidelity to the original model—has received special emphasis. The Learning Collaborative of the Connecticut Center for Effective Practice (CCEP) was chosen to replicate the Child FIRST model. The process has included development of a comprehensive training curriculum and publication of a training manual. Beyond that, however, replication inevitably involves lots of interaction between experienced Child FIRST clinicians and their new colleagues. "Training new staff is intensive and very hands-on," says Darcy Lowell. "There is lots of role playing, lots of discussion. We find that if we can integrate active participation into the training, it's much more effective, and a lot more fun. We have a lot of sharing between teams, so that everyone gets to know one another."

Not surprisingly, clinicians from the various sites describe their work in very similar terms, and the process of sharing among the teams in different cities is ongoing, whether or not training is taking place. Care coordinators also network with one another. In particular they share information about newfound resources they have located. This aspect of the work has become increasingly important and more challenging as state and local budgets have shrunk.

Although the randomized trial has concluded and the study has been published, Child FIRST is continuing to monitor data from all its venues to ensure that outcomes are consistent across the board. Thus far, results achieved at replication sites are similar to those from Bridgeport.

A key goal of the program was met when the federal Health Resources and Services Administration and the Administration for Children and Families designated Child FIRST as one of nine "evidence-based home visiting models" in the country. This designation allows Child FIRST programs to tap into the $1.5 billion in federal funding provided by the Patient Protection and Affordable Care Act. Child FIRST Bridgeport became the first home-based psychotherapeutic intervention for very young children allowed to bill for Medicaid reimbursement in Connecticut.

In January 2012, the Robert Wood Johnson Foundation awarded Child FIRST a grant of $2.3 million for the second phase of its statewide replication. Preparations are under way for the implementation of Child FIRST in New Britain, Middletown, Stamford, and Windham County. As of June 2012, training of clinicians and care coordinators for these venues was complete.

The phase-two grant, which is expected to extend through December 2013, will not only expand Child FIRST operations into these additional venues, but is also expected to facilitate the meshing of the Child FIRST model into the Department of Children and Families. This may happen very quickly. The federal Maternal, Infant, and Early Childhood Home Visiting Program has awarded Connecticut funding that can be used to accelerate establishment of a Child FIRST presence in all fifteen DCF regions in Connecticut.

—⁓— Looking Ahead

Child FIRST is now actively exploring expansion beyond Connecticut. "We are getting many calls from other states," says Lowell. "There is a lot of interest. I expect that in the next year or two, we will see some replication outside of Connecticut."

The completion of the business plan will be one key component of this expansion. The availability of mental health professionals qualified to work with very young children and their families is another factor, and Lowell acknowledges that skilled clinicians can be hard to find. "We need clinicians experienced with children and families who have the right kind of heart," she says. "We look for nurturers—people who care about relationships, and about what goes on inside a parent, and inside a child. We are not looking for people who think they can stop a behavior and solve the problem."

A third factor will be the change that Child FIRST is likely to bring to the large and cumbersome government bureaucracies currently dealing with very young at-risk children at the state and federal levels. Because Child FIRST is so different from the way government agencies have been coping with the problem, adopting Child FIRST as the preferred approach brings with it the potential need to restructure, transform, and even reinvent child welfare agencies.

Connecticut is in the early stages of dealing with this issue. "Child FIRST really challenges a whole lot about the way child protective services operate across the country," says Janice Gruendel, deputy commissioner of the Connecticut Department of Children and Families. "It doesn't just change the world for children—in a positive way; it changes and challenges the way we think about abuse, about neglect, about family-child relationships. Child FIRST pushes us to rethink how we're doing everything, which is a good thing, but a hard thing. It has the potential to challenge governmental child protective systems to be something that they are not right now."

Bureaucratic challenges aside, the advantages of adopting the Child FIRST model are compelling. Some of the advantages are financial. The cost-benefit analysis funded by the Robert Wood Johnson Foundation showed that Child FIRST interventions result in significant governmental savings in the fields of special education, child protective services, foster care, and juvenile justice. The cost of a Child FIRST intervention averages about $6,500 per family.[7] The alternatives are far more expensive. Older children with serious psychological and behavioral issues may be referred by the DCF to Level 2 group homes. A Level 2 group home has 24-hour nursing coverage, and has been described as "one step down from a mental hospital." The cost to the state is just under $100,000 a year per child. DCF places children with violent or criminal tendencies in the state's juvenile training school (aka reform school) at Middletown. If a Level 2 group home is one step down from a mental hospital, the juvenile training school is one step down from prison. The cost of keeping a child incarcerated there exceeds $450,000 a year. A year of inpatient psychiatric hospitalization costs $920,000.

State legislators, public administrators, and budget analysts can do the math. Even in a time of extreme state budget cutbacks, Connecticut found a way to fund Child FIRST. "The science is irrefutable and everybody knows it," says Gruendel. "All of us want every vulnerable child to be competent, capable, and resilient. We want them to be on target with their schooling, their health, and their behaviors in the way they engage with other people. If we truly want all kids to be like our own kids and grandkids, the bottom line is that we don't have a choice. Every day, these at-risk children get one day older."

"These are the children that we as a society give up on, the children we throw away," says Darcy Lowell. "And they end up being the most expensive. These are the kids who have had four pregnancies by the time they're sixteen, who are not literate, who drop out. They end up in foster care or in residential treatment for psychiatric problems, or in the juvenile justice system." The ultimate goal of Child FIRST is to segue from remediation into prevention—to identify at-risk children *before* they display aggressive or disturbed behaviors, language delay, or other psychological problems. "If we can get in there early, we have a good chance of breaking the generational cycle of at-risk kids," Lowell says. "Those children will eventually be different with their own children. Our goal is to support them now so that they grow up with their brains and bodies strong and healthy. They will be better grown-ups and better parents."

—⁓— Epilogue

There is a happy ending to the story of the little boy we started with. Today, he is doing well. His breakthrough came after a Child FIRST team helped his mother deal with her depression, and helped him finally express his hurt and fear—in words rather than through actions. He eventually confronted his father during a prison visit, telling him how angry he was about what he had done. After that, the vomiting stopped. The father was released on parole and reunited with his wife and family. He is supporting his family. The little boy is back in school and thriving. He is also the proud and loving brother to a new baby in the family.

Notes

1. See Begley, S. and Hearn, R. P. "Children's Health Initiatives." *To Improve Health and Health Care 2001: The Robert Wood Johnson Foundation Anthology.* San Francisco: Jossey-Bass, 2001.

2. *Forbes Magazine.* "America's Ten Most Unequal Cities," www.forbes.com/2009/11/30/americas-most-unequal-cities-business-beltway-unequal-cities_slide_2.html.

3. Fraiberg, S., Adelson, E., and Shapiro, V. "Ghosts in the Nursery: A Psychoanalytic Approach to the Problems of Impaired Infant-Mother Relationships." Journal of the American Academy of Child & Adolescent Psychiatry, 1975, *14*, 387–421.

4. See for example Shonkoff, J. P. and Phillips, D. A. (eds.). Committee on Integrating the Science of Early Childhood Development, Board on Children, Youth, and Families, National Research Council and Institute of Medicine, *From Neurons to Neighborhoods: The Science of Early Childhood Development*. Washington, DC: National Academy Press, 2000.

5. Center on the Developing Child. *Toxic Stress: The Facts*, http://developingchild.harvard.edu/topics/science_of_early_childhood/toxic_stress_response/.

6. Lowell, D. I., Carter, A. S., Godoy, L., Paulicin, B., and Briggs-Gowan, M. "A Randomized Controlled Trial of Child FIRST: A Comprehensive Home-Based Intervention Translating Research into Early Childhood Practice." *Child Development*, January/February 2011, *82*(1), 193–208.

7. *Child FIRST Overview*. Unpublished internal Child FIRST document, October 12, 2011.

CHAPTER 13

County Health Rankings & Roadmaps

Irene M. Wielawski

Editors' Introduction

It is no exaggeration to describe the Robert Wood Johnson Foundation as a data-driven organization. There is an inherent belief in the value of good data. The importance of data is illustrated by the many surveys the Foundation has funded to measure such things as access to and quality of care and the percentages of people who smoke, are uninsured, or are overweight. The Foundation has developed quantitative indicators of program results, and it conducts a statistical analysis that measures its own performance as presented in a "scorecard."

But it would be a mistake to conclude that the Foundation cares about data only for its own sake. Rather, the Foundation tends to collect and disseminate data as a way of informing policy and improving programs—thus the great importance given to communicating the results of surveys and studies and of putting them in easily understandable language. The series of Cover the Uninsured Week campaigns is perhaps the most telling example of using data to inform public policy and raise the public's consciousness.

In this chapter, Irene Wielawski, a veteran health care journalist and frequent contributor to the *Anthology* series, explores a new and important source of data, the County Health Rankings, and examines the way in which they are used, especially through the County Health Roadmaps, to encourage local policies that can improve the community's health. In a sense, the County Health Rankings & Roadmaps merge the Foundation's long-standing interest in good data with its newer interest in activities to improve the health of entire populations and communities. And, as Wielawski observes, the County Health Rankings have, in fact, spurred action to improve population health at the local level—either directly through interventions that encourage better health or indirectly through job creation and economic development.

T he Rosedale section of Kansas City, Kansas, in Wyandotte County, shows many signs of a neighborhood that has seen better days—broken sidewalks, houses needing paint, boarded-up storefronts, and empty lots. But there are also bright spots—evidence of a community pulling together to turn things around. Vegetable gardens sprout in some of the vacant lots. Bike paths are being built. And newly poured concrete sidewalks near some elementary schools make it possible for children to walk safely to and from school.

Wendy Wilson, executive director of the Rosedale Development Association since 1993 and a self-described "old hippie," is the driving force behind many of these revitalizing efforts in her ethnically diverse neighborhood of fourteen thousand people. A petite woman with short steel-gray hair and a no-nonsense demeanor, Wilson sees each project as part of the "interconnected" mosaic of community life: If families don't have nourishing food, their health will suffer along with their ability to work and learn. If schools are substandard, children will be handicapped in qualifying for higher education. If a community looks rundown, it will have a harder time attracting new business. And if there are no new businesses, residents will be deprived of services and potential employment.

This holistic view of community life is reflected in the mission of the Rosedale Development Association, described on its website as "policy influencing and advocacy, land use planning, housing construction, crime reduction, public space improvement, youth programming, supporting neighborhood associations and providing assistance to residents and businesses for a host of issues and concerns."[1]

Unfortunately, few of the government programs and philanthropies that Wilson and the Association have turned to for support over the years shared that vision. "Most of them seemed to look at things piecemeal," Wilson said. "They'd see dilapidated buildings and want to fund a housing program, thinking that would fix the community. But, of course, it can't—not by itself."

In the Rosedale Development Association's cramped store-front office on Southwest Boulevard, Wilson and her staff of four young community workers began to doubt that their way of seeing things would ever be embraced by the national agenda setters. And then, in 2010, they were swept up into a countywide planning process stimulated by a program of the Robert Wood Johnson Foundation.

Called "County Health Rankings & Roadmaps," the program uses health and demographic data analyzed by the University of Wisconsin Population Health Institute to score the healthiness of every county in each of the fifty states. The process essentially turns out a report card for each county that identifies strengths in the population, such as low rates of smoking or obesity, and weaknesses, such as high rates of unemployment or births to teenagers. The most striking message of these report cards is the relatively small role played by medical services. Timely access to affordable and high-quality health care—the factors emphasized in the long-running U.S. debate on health reform—account for only about 20 percent of a community's health. Of far greater influence are social, environmental, and behavioral factors such as poverty, violent crime, poor nutrition, inadequate education, and physical inactivity. "I read their report on my county," says Wilson, "and thought, 'Wow, the Robert Wood Johnson Foundation gets it!'"

—⁂— Resetting the Conversation about Health

In fact, the link between health and how we live was not a new discovery for the Robert Wood Johnson Foundation when it set out to expand the work of the University of Wisconsin Population Health Institute into a comprehensive fifty-state ranking system. The Foundation has long been aware of the importance of so-called social determinants of health. As far back as 1972, in his first annual report as the Foundation's president, David Rogers wrote that even though the Foundation was going to focus on improving medical care, he recognized that "while there are serious inequities in available health care, the same is true in other major aspects of our national life, such as housing, nutrition, education, and employment. All of these contribute in important ways to health, or lack of it ... many of our most lethal illnesses stem from the ways in which we use automobiles, alcohol, and drugs, or neglect our bodies; these illnesses are not susceptible to medical intervention working in isolation from other sectors of society."[2]

Nor is the relationship of environment and lifestyle to health a novel concept for public health experts who for centuries have documented these connections—contaminated water supplies, unsanitary hospital conditions, spitting on the sidewalk, lack of mosquito netting, crowded tenements—and, when remedies became available, have pushed for government and civic action. An example is the swift adoption by most countries of lifesaving vaccines once they proved safe for young children. Not only health professionals led the charge for mass vaccination; government and education officials also helped by making vaccines available at low or no cost and mandating them for school enrollment. This collaborative approach greatly accelerated public acceptance of a scientific breakthrough and resulted in millions of people being saved from disability and premature death.

Less obvious—but no less critical to population health—are the myriad collaborations between government and the private sector on issues that many people would consider outside the medical realm. Take road safety, for example. From decisions by municipal highway departments on where to locate traffic lights, crosswalks, and speed bumps to choices made by automobile manufacturers on such things as chassis materials, airbag release points, crumple zone design, and seatbelt locks, each rests on a foundation of concern for public safety.

This collaborative commitment frayed somewhat during the 1980s, 1990s, and early 2000s as the national conversation about health became focused on affordability. Patrick Remington, professor and associate dean at the University of Wisconsin School of Medicine and Public Health, recalls how even physicians lost sight of their historic role as civic leaders on health matters. "As health care became more of a business enterprise," he says, "and as health care leaders saw businessmen taking over, there was a tremendous push for physicians to get MBAs in order to qualify as administrative leaders." Suddenly, it seemed smart for physicians to view their practices as business enterprises oriented solely to the needs of paying "customers." Traditional but often unpaid community service roles such as being the team doctor at school athletic events or volunteering in a free clinic for the poor took a back seat. Among employers, the conversation turned to strategies on ways to discourage the use of health benefits or increase workers' share of the insurance premium. In policy and political circles, the focus was on how to cover the growing number of Americans without health insurance and not break the bank.

The trend dismayed Remington and others in the public health field who knew the limits of medical science to fix most people's health problems. Clinicians—even those scrambling to add MBA to the MD or RN after their names—knew this as well through their daily interactions with patients. The reason for the visit might be fatigue or insomnia, but the larger context—a patient's fifty extra pounds, the six-pack-a-night habit, hounding creditors—often mattered more from a health standpoint and influenced treatment decisions. "The fact that we have high rates of unemployment, children in poverty, smoking, and obesity that affect health is not a surprise to physicians," says Remington. "But during this period physicians stopped feeling they had community responsibility or accountability for these social conditions."

—⁓— From Global Snapshots to Local Action

Most people don't think or talk about their health in the crisp terms of a business school case study. They use emotional and unscientific phrases like "I'm not myself" and "I'm stressed out" even when seeking help for overtly clinical symptoms like back spasms or digestive problems. The failures of their bodies are inseparable from the larger tableau of their lives, including social and environmental conditions. Global health studies support this view of health as more than personal biology, documenting, for example, significantly shorter lifespans in countries with inadequate health care systems, unchecked infectious disease, contaminated water, and ongoing warfare.

Although they illuminate the larger context of health, these global snapshots give little guidance on what people living in these places actually can do about unhealthful conditions. The scale is too large. Breaking down the data by county helps somewhat, but the focus is still too diffuse to stimulate citizen action. In the United States, for example, a project of the United Health Foundation, in collaboration with the American Public Health Association and the Partnership for Prevention, called *America's Health Rankings*, has compiled health-related data for each of the fifty states every year since 1990. It's a popular story with the media, but only a handful of states have significantly improved their standings—notably Vermont which climbed from seventeenth place in 1998 to first place in 2010.[3]

By contrast, Mississippi and other poor southern states such as Louisiana, Arkansas, and Alabama remain glued to the bottom, with Mississippi coming in last for ten years straight. That track record has bred a sort of gallows humor among health officials in the persistently low-scoring states. "Thank God for Mississippi," they say every time their own state ekes out a ranking just shy of worst in the nation. The quip barely masks the frustration of trying to make headway against myriad local health-undermining conditions within the bare-bones budgets of chronically poor states. What's needed is local buy-in. But to get that requires greater public understanding about health and its disparate influences, and a better tool to identify and remedy unhealthy conditions than existing big-picture snapshots like *America's Health Rankings* or the massive state and federal government data sets utilized primarily by researchers.

Against this backdrop, the University of Wisconsin's Public Health and Health Policy Institute (the name was changed in 2005 to Population Health Institute) decided in the early 2000s to devise a more locally relevant statistical snapshot. The idea was to present selected data in the larger context of socioeconomic and behavioral health influences so that people could see not only the level of health in their communities but also the contributing environmental and socioeconomic conditions. The goal was to help community leaders see their inherent role in safeguarding public health.

"We specifically picked health access and affordability," says Remington, who at the time was director of the institute, located within the University of Wisconsin-Madison School of Medicine and Public Health. "But we also picked behaviors and employment rates and children staying in school and so on." Remington's research team decided to work off the *America's Health Rankings* model and adapt it to Wisconsin's counties. To show the interrelationships between people's health and their lifestyles and living conditions, the researchers merged traditional health "outcomes" information such as life span and rates of disease with so-called health "determinant" information such as rates of tobacco and alcohol use and physical inactivity. The "determinants" factors were categorized this way:

- Access to medical care, including whether people had health insurance, regular dental care, and blood pressure checks
- Health behaviors, including tobacco use, physical activity, consumption of fruits and vegetables, incidence of sexually transmitted diseases, and so on
- Socioeconomic factors, including the high school graduation rate and household income

- The physical environment, such as air and water quality and lead levels*

The County Health Rankings that emerged gave equal weight to the factors contributing to the quality of people's health, including the consequences of living with chronic illnesses such as diabetes, as they did to premature death (statistically measured as "years of potential life lost"). "Health outcomes are often reported in terms of mortality, since years of life is very important and mortality data are available and reliable," Remington and colleagues explained in their debut report, *Wisconsin County Health Rankings, 2003*. "However, most of us believe that health is measured not only in years of life but also in the quality of those years. Thus, we have created a health outcome ranking that incorporates how people in Wisconsin communities rate the state of their health while alive."[4]

Wisconsin's experiment wasn't an overnight success. Some critics questioned the statistical legitimacy of comparing sparsely populated rural counties against densely populated metropolitan counties with plentiful resources but also greater infrastructure costs and socioeconomic diversity. The feedback stimulated refinement of the model. "We got complaints, we made changes," Remington says. And the researchers frankly acknowledged in the report cards that some of the data upon which the rankings were based was several years old, albeit the best available. This disclosure was characteristic of the pull-no-punches style of the report cards,

---

* The original Wisconsin Health Rankings in 2003 attributed 10 percent of health status to access to medical care; 40 percent to behavioral factors; 40 percent to socioeconomic factors; and 10 percent to the physical environment. Upon a further review of the literature after the scope of the program became national, the Institute revised the formula to accord with the latest findings. It attributed 20 percent of health status to medical care; 30 percent to behavioral factors; 40 percent to socioeconomic factors; and 10 percent to the physical environment.

which were aimed at forging a respectful dialogue and partnership with community leaders who were engaged in a difficult task.

From Wisconsin's counties came glimmers of response. One county, with grant support from the American Academy of Pediatrics, started a program in which at every doctor's visit young children receive a book to take home and read with their parents—an activity considered by child health experts to be important for emotional development and school readiness. Another county, in a rural part of the state, responded to damning statistics on dental health and inappropriate emergency room use by partnering with the local hospital to open a sliding fee–scale medical and dental clinic for people without health insurance.

"The rankings aren't the be-all and end-all, but they're a conversation starter and they get people working on things," says Remington.

—ᴡᴡ— Taking the Conversation National

In 2008, Remington and his team approached the Robert Wood Johnson Foundation for a modest grant that would enable the University of Wisconsin Population Health Institute to expand the Wisconsin model to five additional states. Instead, the Foundation offered nearly $5 million so the Institute could produce report cards for every county in every state—a total of three thousand counties.[5]

James Marks, a leading expert on disease prevention who joined the Foundation in 2004 as senior vice president in charge of health, championed the fifty-state push. The evidence from Wisconsin suggested that giving communities the tools to identify their own health disparities might yield more comprehensive and sustained attention than grant-funded, single-issue initiatives. A fifty-state archive of county report cards also had a better chance of creating national awareness of the so-called social determinants of health than experiments in a few scattered states. Furthermore, Marks believed the report cards had the potential to spur broad-based action to reduce health disparities among

Americans—a problem the Foundation had long considered a funding priority.

Marks also shared Remington's view that the national conversation about health had become overly focused on cost and affordability, creating a false public message that health could be bought with an insurance card. That, in turn, allowed people like doctors and hospital executives, mayors, school superintendents, and business and religious leaders to withdraw from their previously embraced obligations to address unhealthy conditions in their communities. "Too many Americans are dying young and too many people say they don't feel well," says Marks. "This is not the fault of health departments or the health care system nor is it solely their job to fix these problems. It's an obligation for all of us to contribute to health."

The Foundation saw the Wisconsin model as more than just an educational tool for those seeking to understand the roots of ill health in their communities. It also had the potential to be a powerful social-messaging vehicle to, in Marks' words, "galvanize action" by elected officials and other community leaders. Hence the importance of ranking counties from best to worst in their respective states, and breaking out specific data to show civic leaders where they were beating state averages and where they were falling down on the job. The Foundation hoped to stimulate people's competitive instincts while also helping them identify health problems that could reasonably be tackled and, over time, reduced. The theory was that success in achieving a higher rank or ameliorating a specific problem would provide the psychic boost needed to keep going on problems as entrenched as obesity, substance abuse, and crime. In this way, the annual report card might play a role similar to that of the giant United Way thermometer displayed during community fundraising campaigns. Each uptick toward the top helps stimulate a collective sense of accomplishment and recharges enthusiasm for reaching the goal.

In October 2008, the Foundation authorized County Health Rankings: Mobilizing Action Toward Community Health (MATCH), providing roughly $5 million through August 2012 to pay for three successive annual rankings. The Population Health Institute issued the County Health Rankings in 2010, 2011, and 2012, and the Foundation assisted with a sophisticated media campaign, including creation of an easy-to-use public website showcasing the report cards and supporting research; instructional webinars on social change strategies; press conferences; and promotional videos on communities working to improve local health conditions.

Two years later, in October 2010, the Foundation made a $15 million commitment to follow up on its initial investment in County Health Rankings by adding a program called County Health Roadmaps. Headed by Bridget Booske Catlin, a colleague of Remington at the University of Wisconsin, County Health Roadmaps enabled the Population Health Institute to build on the momentum created by the County Health Rankings by supporting, with two-year grants totaling up to $200,000 (with a required match of cash and in-kind services), up to thirty-two counties and communities taking action to improve the social, behavioral, and environmental conditions that undermine health. (The Foundation added $1.3 million in 2012 for the grants program.) In addition, the Roadmaps program provides support for a new center providing technical assistance to communities around the country (not just those funded by the Roadmaps program), for new partnerships with national organizations such as United Way, and for an annual prize that recognizes communities for their outstanding work to improve health.

"It's not good enough to tell people to take walks outside when they live in a dangerous neighborhood, or to eat fresh fruits and vegetables if there is no supermarket nearby," says Brenda Henry, a senior research and evaluation officer at the Foundation. "The Roadmaps initiative is intended to put our money where our mouth is and help communities devise strategies to move the needle on community improvement."

To assist communities as they plan and implement their strategies, the Foundation commissioned Community Catalyst, a

Boston-based national advocacy organization, to provide technical assistance to the communities selected. The projects range widely, from efforts to help ex-convicts reenter their communities, to improved transit systems, to preschool programs, to business coalitions working toward local job creation. The thread that binds them to County Health Rankings is that they in some way target what researchers consider to be the social determinants of poor health.

Abbey Cofsky, the Foundation program officer in charge of County Health Rankings & Roadmaps, acknowledges the long and difficult road to turning around health-eroding personal behaviors and socioeconomic conditions. "We don't expect to transform health outcomes with two-year grants," Cofsky says. "But we do see County Health Rankings & Roadmaps projects as a way to change how community leaders invest time and resources. And they are critically important steps towards gaining better public understanding of health—notably that how well we feel and how long we live are influenced by factors outside the health care system."

So where has it led? The most measurable result has been in media coverage. The Foundation's Marks says the first fifty-state County Health Rankings report generated thousands of print, radio, and television reports. And for a brief moment, the report actually made it to the top of the hit parade on the search engine Google. It's harder to measure the response—and the quality of response—from the counties themselves. Some haven't done anything to speak of. Others leaped to examine their problems and strategize about solutions. Still others saw activity by smaller units within the county—a city, perhaps, or a school system—to address a single factor with implications for people's long-term health.

Following are two examples of action spurred, in part, by the County Health Rankings & Roadmaps initiative. The problems spotlighted in the data categories were, for the most part, already known. But in one case, Wyandotte County, Kansas, the mayor swung the report card like a billy club to get people around the table who had never worked together on a common task. In the other, Hampden County, Massachusetts, an existing community health coalition in the depressed city of Springfield got a boost toward a long-cherished jobs project to alleviate urban unemployment.

⎯⤳⎯ Wyandotte County, Kansas

Remember Wendy Wilson? She's the community activist stubbornly applying "old hippie" thinking to improve life in down-at-the-heels Rosedale. Rosedale, in turn, is part of Kansas City, Kansas, which is the dominant city in Wyandotte County, located just across the Missouri River from the better-known Kansas City, Missouri. There are only two other municipalities in Wyandotte County, Bonner Springs and Edwardsville, both small towns. Because of this, Kansas City, Kansas, and the county operate in a unified government structure. The city's mayor, Joe Reardon, is also Wyandotte County CEO, which means that everything—good and bad—that happens in the county's 156 square miles lands on his desk.

The first health rankings, released in August 2009, were actually a precursor to the national version, which was rolled out a year later. Kansas was one of a handful of states that used the Wisconsin model to independently rank their own counties. When the results were in, Wyandotte sat at the bottom of Kansas's 105 counties. The health rankings arrived in Wyandotte County amid a hailstorm of bad news. Already economically depressed from a steady decline in meatpacking jobs, Wyandotte was reeling from the ripple effects of a national recession that showed no signs of abating. Bankruptcies and foreclosures were at record levels and property values had plummeted—triggering a vicious cycle of reduced tax revenue and corresponding reductions in government services just when people needed them most. For Wyandotte County to be publicly spotlighted as the least healthy county in the entire state of Kansas was, to say the least, a stunning new challenge to Reardon's four-year-old administration. He decided to meet it head on.

"There's a moment in time for a political official and this was mine," says Reardon. "I simply had to own the rankings even though the problems that were identified had been with us for a long time and I knew it was going to be very difficult to change our ranking in short order."

Caitlin McMurtry, a policy analyst at the Kansas Health Institute that did the 2009 ranking analysis, recalls the phone call she got from an exercised Joe Reardon, summoning her to Kansas City. McMurtry's sit-down with Reardon was the beginning of an ambitious, two-year research and planning process called Healthy Communities Wyandotte. County health director Joe Connor remembers how widely—and how passionately—opinions ranged during the early meetings at City Hall. Everyone seemed to have an opinion on how to solve Wyandotte's health problems. There certainly were a lot to choose from. Wyandotte County exceeds both Kansas and national norms for smoking, obesity, and sexually transmitted infections. Its teen birth rate is twice that of the Kansas rate and more than three times the national rate. Joblessness and the percentage of uninsured residents are higher than the U.S. rates, and preventable hospital stays exceed both Kansas and national benchmarks.

But mostly, Connor remembers the mayor's parting words at the kickoff meeting: "Oh, by the way, Joe Connor's going to lead this."

Connor was the logical choice, of course. As director of the Wyandotte County/Kansas City Public Health Department, he already supervised public and environmental health, air quality, and emergency preparedness. He was also known for his organizational acumen, which played out in Healthy Communities Wyandotte through the formation of five actions teams: communications, education, environmental infrastructure, nutrition, and health services.

Political observers identify another factor in his selection: Connor's stature as a true "son of the Dotte." Like Mayor Reardon, Connor grew up in Kansas City, Kansas, had family connections throughout the county, and regularly stepped up as a volunteer in schools, community organizations, and at church. As for the charismatic Reardon, not only is he one of the youngest mayors in the city's history, he's also the son of the late Jack Reardon, a popular civic leader, mayor from 1975 to 1987, and namesake of Kansas City's Jack Reardon Convention Center. Between them, Connor and Reardon were able to corral just about every community leader necessary to bring credibility, practical know-how, and political clout to the undertaking.

The capstone was their recruitment of Barbara Atkinson, who was then the executive vice chancellor of the University of Kansas Medical Center, one of the largest employers in Wyandotte County and seat of the state medical school. "The fact that Barbara Atkinson, Joe Connor, and Mayor Reardon teamed up and came to every meeting, that's what sold me," says Martha Staker, director of Project EAGLE, a program for infants and preschool children considered at risk for health and learning problems. Staker ended up chairing the Education for a Healthy Community action team.

Collectively, team members committed hundreds of hours of personal time to hone ideas for health-enhancing community projects and related policy revisions. Staker's team, for example, worked on a system of incentives to reduce Wyandotte County's 40 percent high school dropout rate. The County Health Rankings report hadn't told educators anything they didn't already know about school dropouts, but viewing the dropout problem in the context of other Kansas counties and statewide trends helped spur the community to take action.

"We're a blue-collar town, meaning a lot of our kids come from families that did not necessarily finish high school but still had good-paying jobs in the meatpacking plants," says Reardon. "Well, the world's changed. We have a meat slicing plant that

Sara Lee opened here recently with two hundred jobs. But the entire plant is computerized—no human hands touch the meat! Our kids need different skills from their parents and it's our job to prepare them."

Action team leaders recruited people they thought had the professional expertise and practical wisdom to shape ideas into recommendations for action or policy change. Wendy Wilson was tapped for the Healthy Food action team, which eventually got behind a recommendation for zoning restrictions so that fast-food restaurants couldn't have drive-through service in residential areas. This was primarily to eliminate danger to pedestrians from cars zipping in and out, but the recommendation also dovetailed with the sidewalk construction projects under way to encourage walking to school and elsewhere. Wilson was thrilled to see her ideal of holistic neighborhood planning being embraced by others, but she also came to realize that teammates had been thinking similarly all along. "Working on the team introduced me to people who could be allies for our work in Rosedale," says Wilson.

Bob Van Maren, superintendent of the Bonner Springs-Edwardsville school district, likewise met potential collaborators through his work on the Education for a Healthy Community team. "I've become more aware of what other people are doing in the community and how we can help each other," he says.

Among the goals endorsed by the action teams are dental care clinics; school policies to foster nutritious eating habits in children; a nurse home-visiting program; training and deployment of community health workers; after-school mentoring projects; mental health outreach; a countywide communication initiative to educate people about healthy living; tax credits for farm produce vendors; and training programs to promote cultural competence.

This last goal came about through the influence of Mary Lou Jaramillo, president and CEO of El Centro, a social service agency relied upon by the county's growing Spanish-speaking population. Jaramillo insisted that an El Centro representative sit on every action team to make sure the needs of Latino residents were incorporated into the new initiatives. She recalled the chaos that erupted in the Latino community when Kansas state school authorities adopted a "no exceptions" policy to its school immunization requirement. "We had some new immigrant families who simply weren't familiar with immunization," she says. "They don't take their children to the doctor unless they are sick. Their children were barred on the first day of school, and suddenly we had all those parents coming to El Centro, very upset."

In response, El Centro launched programs to train neighborhood women to be *promotoras de salud*—community health educators—to explain things like immunization requirements and the reasons for preventive care such as prenatal and well-baby checkups. Through the action teams, Jaramillo hoped to integrate her agency's specialized programs with those of the health department and other agencies so Latino families could benefit from municipal offerings such as blood-pressure screenings, flu shots, and other health and wellness programs.

The work of the action teams officially ended in December 2011, when Healthy Communities Wyandotte delivered its report on goals and priorities to Mayor Reardon and shared it with county residents on the health department's webpage. There was a brief euphoric feeling of accomplishment—followed by a huge letdown.

The precipitating event was the Foundation's rejection of Wyandotte County's application for a Roadmaps grant. County officials had been confident of getting a grant because of the Foundation's demonstrated enthusiasm for the planning process undertaken by Healthy Communities Wyandotte—including sending a camera crew to film action team meetings and featuring the video on websites promoting the County Health Rankings project.

The failure to get a Roadmaps grant came as a shock that undercut momentum and spawned second-guessing. "What did we do wrong?" people wondered. The grant was seen as crucial to launching projects that could sustain popular interest in tackling health threats. The fact remains that many of these threats correlate with poverty, and Wyandotte is one of the poorest counties in Kansas, a state whose own coffers are depleted by national recession. Where, people asked, was the capital for health coaches and new mental health services and after-school mentoring and more sidewalks to come from?

Ever practical, as civic leaders in hard-up communities tend to be, Wyandotte's political leaders are now eyeing "community contribution" revenue from a new casino in the western part of the county. An estimated $2 million will become available to the Wyandotte/Kansas City Unified Government in January 2014. If Mayor Reardon is still in office (the reelection contest is in 2013), he says he plans to push hard for Healthy Communities projects. But he needs a majority vote by county commissioners and notes that some of them have already suggested alternative investments.

Barbara Atkinson, the former University of Kansas Medical School executive who helped lead the planning process, remains foursquare behind the recommendations. As a pathologist and longtime champion of partnerships between the medical school and county health projects, she did not need County Health Rankings to teach her the complexities of population health. But Atkinson is concerned about leaning too hard on a strategy that employs fear of ill health to power efforts to ameliorate what most people see as poverty-related conditions.

"I think it's a hard sell and can make people jaded," Atkinson says, noting that even the term *public health* implies *welfare* to some people. She hopes that early funding goes to projects to help Wyandotte's youngsters avoid early pregnancy and, at minimum, attain a high school diploma. In her judgment, tangible and timely results are more likely to result from such education-related initiatives than from efforts to reduce the rates of smoking, alcohol abuse, and obesity. Corresponding improvement in the employment opportunities for Wyandotte's young people will, Atkinson believes, help to sell longer-term investments in population health.

"The money commitment has to be long term in order to measure results or progress," says Atkinson. "We can't be fighting for renewal every year."

—⌇— Hampden County, Massachusetts

Based on the analysis by County Health Rankings, Hampden County, Massachusetts, and Wyandotte County, Kansas, could be twins—albeit 1,400 miles apart.

Compared to other counties in their respective states and to some national benchmarks, their scores are terrible. Each has nearly double the U.S. unemployment rate. They have more violent crime in their communities than other places do, more births to teenage mothers, more single-parent homes, and a higher percentage of people who report feeling unwell, physically and mentally. The combination of these factors portends significant long-term health problems and shorter life spans if residents fail to turn things around.

The difference is in how community leaders have responded to the report cards. Where Wyandotte dug into each data category and spent two years developing a multipronged plan to remedy health hazards, Hampden boiled everything down to a single goal: *more jobs*.

Health is explicitly *not* the driver of activities currently being supported by a two-year Roadmaps grant of roughly $200,000 a year to Hampden County. There are some health care players, notably the two major health systems in the region, Baystate Health and the Sisters of Providence Health System. But their participation has as much to do with their business interests in Hampden County as with their health care mission.

The other difference is the focus of the project. It is centered exclusively on the city of Springfield and, more specifically, on neighborhoods where county-level health statistics don't even begin to describe the hazards of living there. "The County Health Rankings are really a poverty map," says Frank Robinson, who wears two hats in the Hampden County venture. One is as director of community health planning for the region's major hospital, Baystate Medical Center. The other is as executive director of a business coalition called Partners for a Healthier Community, which successfully competed for a Roadmaps grant. "Bad as Hampden County looks, the conditions in some neighborhoods in Springfield are grossly worse," Robinson says. "The rankings kind of wash out the true picture of our population's needs."

This merger of local wisdom with the County Health Rankings report card has prompted an economic development push called the Wellspring Initiative. Modeled on the successful Evergreen Cooperatives in Cleveland, Ohio, Wellspring is seeking to create new businesses to compete for service contracts—and jobs—that Springfield's anchor institutions are currently outsourcing to distant vendors. Among the enterprises under consideration is a commercial laundry that could serve the needs of local hospitals, colleges, nursing homes, and other institutions. Also under discussion is a fresh food distribution hub, through which fruits and vegetables would be purchased from local growers and sold to institutional clients.

In addition to the Baystate and Sisters of Providence health systems, Wellspring's backers include the Center for Public Policy and Administration and the Center for Popular Economics at the University of Massachusetts, Amherst; several local colleges and universities; community partners such as Jobs with Justice, Pioneer Valley AFL-CIO, and the New North Citizens Council, a social service agency in one of Springfield's most distressed neighborhoods; and funding partners such as the MassMutual Foundation and the United Way of Pioneer Valley. The project's technical advisers include the Federal Reserve Bank of Boston, which deploys economic data much in the way the University of Wisconsin Population Health Institute uses health statistics to create the County Health Rankings. A Wellspring report based in part on the bank's 2010 report, titled *Jobs in Springfield,*

Massachusetts: Understanding and Remedying the Causes of Low Resident Employment Rates,[6] starkly laid out the case for more jobs:

- Annual household income in Springfield's poorest neighborhoods ranged between $15,000 and $17,000, compared to a Massachusetts average of $64,000.

- Of 10,300 jobs in Springfield, only 1,500 are held by Springfield residents due to gaps in education and skills.

- Although anchor institutions in Springfield annually purchase $1.5 billion in goods and services, 90 percent of the contracts go to businesses outside the region.

"Jobs are the key to improving the entire quality of life for our families, including health," says Michael Denney, executive director of the New North Citizens' Council, a social service agency in Springfield's impoverished Memorial Square neighborhood, where the population is largely Latino. "That's why the job focus of Wellspring is really exciting to me. We used to have factory jobs right here in the neighborhood. People could walk to work, walk home for lunch. But the last one left about seven years ago and now all we've got are the McDonald's and the Dunkin' Donuts and that wage scale simply doesn't work when you're trying to support a family. We need good paying jobs with benefits."

Phillip González, the project director for the Roadmaps to Health Community Grants, acknowledges Wellspring's seeming disconnect from the health message of the County Health Rankings. But González, who works for Community Catalyst, which is providing technical assistance under the Roadmaps project, says the Roadmaps portfolio tends toward single-issue projects that relate to health only in the big picture. Besides Wellspring, Roadmaps is funding projects to help children bond with incarcerated parents, prepare young people for school and careers, and improve public transportation.

"Although the Robert Wood Johnson Foundation is a dedicated health funder, that's not the language or strategy we're using in Springfield," says González, adding that civic leaders there pointedly rejected the health message imbedded in the County Health Rankings in order to stay focused on jobs development. "The words to me were just that: 'Our goal is jobs. Our people need a reason to get up and go to work and pay their bills. Of course, we want them to take care of their health, but first they have to have jobs to be able to pay the co-pays on their medicines and actually take them.'"

Ira Rubenzahl, president of Springfield Technical Community College and a Wellspring Initiative partner, says that he grasps the relationship between life circumstances and health outcomes but believes that a focus on jobs creation is a much more powerful way to galvanize community support for social improvements. "People understand that improving employment opportunities means people can be more self-sufficient, neighborhoods will improve, crime will go down, and the city will have more resources to do what it has to do like fix the roads and plow the snow," Rubenzahl says.

He notes an additional motivating force: the economics principle of enlightened self-interest among businesses backing—and potentially investing in—Wellspring enterprises. "The college is involved partly because it's good for our business. More jobs and improvements in the standard of living and local economy mean better health but also less crime and better city services. If the city is so depleted that it can't plow the roads—and that's happened in recent winters—our faculty and students can't get to class. That's bad for my business."

—∾— Conclusion

Pat Remington of the University of Wisconsin Population Health Institute modestly refers to County Health Rankings as a "conversation starter" that might yield measurable improvements in population health a generation from now. The modesty is well placed. So much of what the report cards identify as deleterious to health and life span—adult obesity, alcohol abuse, unemployment—are extremely difficult to turn around in the short term. And, as the snapshots of Wyandotte and Hampden counties show, how local communities respond to their report cards and the type of conversation that ensues vary greatly.

Although the improvements in health may not be seen in the near term, County Health Rankings & Roadmaps has nonetheless been valuable as a means to stimulate public discussion of broader influences on health than simply access or lack of access to medical care. This shift in emphasis has been under way for some time among health policy experts grappling with the soaring costs of treating illness. Within the Robert Wood Johnson Foundation, campaigns to reduce smoking and obesity, community-improvement efforts such as the anti–substance abuse programs Free to Grow and Fighting Back, and support for the Commission to Build a Healthier America manifest this broader perspective on population health. Beyond the work of the Robert Wood Johnson Foundation, it can be seen in provisions tucked into the Affordable Care Act to promote healthy behavior and prevent illness, in school policies to teach children about nutrition, and in workplace wellness programs that encourage employees to eat better, exercise more, and stop smoking.

In this larger context, then, the unique contribution of County Health Rankings & Roadmaps is to share this perspective with local communities, give them the tools to set priorities, and provide support to implement homegrown solutions. Wyandotte County, Kansas, and Hampden County, Massachusetts, show how differently the health message of the Rankings may be received and converted to action. But it's the start of an important conversation.

Notes

1. Rosedale Development Association website, http://rosedale.org.
2. Rogers, D. "The President's Statement." *Robert Wood Johnson Foundation Annual Report 1972*.
3. United Health Foundation. *America's Health Rankings*, http://www.americashealthrankings.org/Rankings.
4. Peppard, P. E. et al. *Wisconsin County Health Rankings, 2003*. Madison: Wisconsin Public Health and Health Policy Institute, 2003, p. 1.
5. RWJF Funding Summary report, funding ID 65017.
6. Kodrzycki, Y. *Jobs in Springfield, Massachusetts: Understanding and Remedying the Causes of Low Resident Employment, Community Affairs Discussion Paper 2009–05*. Boston: Federal Reserve Bank of Boston, 2010.

───ᴍᴍ───The Editors

David C. Colby, PhD, the vice president of research and evaluation at the Robert Wood Johnson Foundation, leads a team dedicated to improving the nation's ability to understand key health and health care issues so that informed decisions can be made concerning the way Americans maintain health and obtain health care. His team also assesses how the Foundation is doing through evaluations, performance measures, and scorecards. He came to the Foundation in January 1998 after nine years of service with the Medicare Payment Advisory Commission and the Physician Payment Review Commission, where he was deputy director. Earlier, he taught at the University of Maryland Baltimore County, Williams College, and State University College at Buffalo. Colby's published research focused on Medicaid and Medicare, use of emergency departments, AIDS, and various topics in political science. He was an associate editor of the *Journal of Health Politics, Policy and Law* from 1995 to 2002. He received his doctorate in political science from the University of Illinois, a master of arts from Ohio University, and a bachelor of arts from Ohio Wesleyan University.

Stephen L. Isaacs, JD, is a partner in Isaacs/Jellinek, a San Francisco–based consulting firm, and president of Health Policy Associates, Inc. A former professor of public health at Columbia University and the founding director of its Development Law and Policy Program, he has written extensively for professional and popular audiences. His book, *The Consumer's Legal Guide to Today's Health Care*, was reviewed as "the single best guide to the health care system in print today." His articles have been syndicated and have appeared in law reviews and health policy journals. He also provides technical assistance internationally on health law, civil society, and social policy. A graduate of Brown University and Columbia Law School, Isaacs served as vice president of the International Planned Parenthood's Western Hemisphere Region, practiced health law, and spent four years in Thailand as a program officer with the U.S. Agency for International Development.

—ᴡᴡ—The Contributors

Will Bunch is the senior writer for the *Philadelphia Daily News* and its former political writer, gaining national recognition for his scoops on 9/11 and the war in Iraq. Before coming to Philadelphia, Bunch was a key member of the New York Newsday team that won the 1992 Pulitzer Prize for spot news reporting. His magazine articles have appeared in a number of national and regional publications, including *The New York Times Magazine*. Bunch is also the author of three books, including *The Backlash: Right-Wing Radicals, High-Def Hucksters, and Paranoid Politics in the Age of Obama* and two recent Kindle Single e-books on Occupy Wall Street and the 1948 NFL championship game.

Digby Diehl is a writer, literary collaborator, and television, print, and Internet journalist. His book credits include *Rather Outspoken*, the bestselling memoir of journalist Dan Rather; *Patti LuPone: A Memoir*, written in collaboration with one of Broadway's foremost leading ladies; *Priceless Memories*, the autobiography of Bob Barker; *Remembering Grace*, a look back at the life of Grace Kelly (with Kay Diehl); *Angel on My Shoulder*, the autobiography of singer Natalie Cole; *The Million Dollar Mermaid*, the autobiography of MGM star Esther Williams; *Tales from the Crypt*, the history of the popular comic book, movie, and television series; and *A Spy for All Seasons*, the autobiography of former CIA officer Duane Clarridge. For eleven years, Diehl was the literary correspondent for ABC-TV's *Good Morning America*, and was the book editor for the *Home Page* show on MSNBC. Previously the entertainment editor for KCBS television in Los Angeles, he was a writer for the Emmys and for the soap opera

Santa Barbara, book editor of the *Los Angeles Herald-Examiner*, editor in chief of art book publisher Harry N. Abrams, and the founding book editor of the *Los Angeles Times Book Review*. Diehl holds an MA in theatre from UCLA and a BA in American studies from Rutgers University, where he was a Henry Rutgers Scholar.

Risa Lavizzo-Mourey, MD, MBA, is the fourth president and CEO of the Robert Wood Johnson Foundation, a position she assumed in January 2003. She originally joined the staff in April 2001 as senior vice president and director, Health Care Group. Prior to coming to the Foundation, Lavizzo-Mourey was the Sylvan Eisman Professor of Medicine and Health Care Systems at the University of Pennsylvania, as well as director of the Institute on Aging. She was the deputy administrator of the Agency for Health Care Policy and Research, now known as the Agency for Healthcare Research and Quality, within the Department of Health and Human Services. While in government service, Lavizzo-Mourey worked on the White House Health Care Policy team, including the White House Task Force on Health Care Reform where she cochaired the working group on Quality of Care. Lavizzo-Mourey has served on many federal advisory committees, including the Task Force on Aging Research; the National Committee for Vital and Health Statistics, where she chaired the Subcommittee on Minority Populations; and the President's Advisory Commission on Consumer Protection and Quality in the Health Care Industry. She recently completed work as codirector of a congressionally requested Institute of Medicine study on racial disparities in health care resulting in the publication of *Unequal Treatment: Confronting Racial and Ethnic Disparities in Health Care*. She is the author of several books and dozens of articles. Lavizzo-Mourey is a member of the Institute of Medicine of the National Academy of Sciences. She is the recipient of eight honorary doctorates and numerous other awards, including those received from the Harvard School of Public Health, Department of Health and Human Services, National Academy of

Sciences, American College of Physicians, National Library of Medicine, American Medical Women's Association, National Medical Association, and University of Pennsylvania. Lavizzo-Mourey earned a medical degree at Harvard Medical School, followed by a master's in business administration at the University of Pennsylvania's Wharton School. After completing a residency in internal medicine at Brigham and Women's Hospital in Boston, she was a Robert Wood Johnson Clinical Scholar at the University of Pennsylvania, where she received her geriatrics training.

Sarah G. Pickell is director of communications and development at the Institute for Advanced Studies in Culture, an interdisciplinary research center and intellectual community at the University of Virginia committed to understanding contemporary cultural change and its individual and social consequences, training young scholars, and providing intellectual leadership in service to the public good. Previously, she worked at the Virginia Foundation for the Humanities and at the Robert Wood Johnson Foundation. As a research assistant for research and evaluation at the Robert Wood Johnson Foundation, her work focused on measuring organizational effectiveness and disseminating findings from research and evaluation grantees. She received a BA in history from the College of William & Mary.

Tony Proscio is a senior fellow at the Center for Strategic Philanthropy and Civil Society at Duke University's Sanford School of Public Policy and a consultant to foundations and major nonprofit organizations. He offers strategic consulting on program design, planning, and evaluation; communication; and policy analysis and development. He is coauthor, with Paul S. Grogan, of the book *Comeback Cities: A Blueprint for Urban Neighborhood Revival*, and has written three essays on civic and philanthropic jargon published by the Edna McConnell Clark Foundation. In the 1990s he was associate editor of the *Miami Herald*, where he was lead editorial writer on economic issues and wrote a weekly opinion column.

Sara Solovitch is a writer whose stories have appeared in *Esquire*, *Wired*, *Outside*, and other publications. She has been a staff reporter at several major newspapers, including the *Philadelphia Inquirer,* and has had numerous stories published in the *Washington Post* and the *Los Angeles Times*. For six years, she wrote a weekly column on children's health for the *San Jose Mercury News*. She is currently at work on her first book, *Please Shoot the Piano Player*, an examination of stage fright, which is slated for publication by Bloomsbury Press in 2014. She lives in Santa Cruz, California.

Irene M. Wielawski is an independent writer and editor specializing in health care and policy topics. She has written extensively on socioeconomic issues in American medicine, particularly the difficulties faced by people without timely access to medical services because of financial, geographic, cultural, and other barriers. Wielawski was a staff writer for nearly twenty years for daily newspapers, most recently the *Los Angeles Times*, where she was a member of the investigations team. Subsequently, with a research grant from the Robert Wood Johnson Foundation, she tracked local efforts to care for the medically uninsured. Other commissioned projects include producing pediatric medicine segments for public television and an analysis of the Massachusetts health reform law. Her independent work appears in *The New York Times, Los Angeles Times*, and *Kaiser Health News* among daily outlets, on websites, and in peer-reviewed journals and books. Wielawski has been a finalist for the Pulitzer Prize for medical reporting and shared in two *Los Angeles Times* staff Pulitzers, among other honors. She is a founder and current board member of the Association of Health Care Journalists, a reviewer for *Health Affairs*, and a graduate of Vassar College.

—ᴡ—Index